JA

MIND.

BODY.

MIRACLE.

Holistic healthy habits and
daily disciplines to miraculously
transform your mind and body.

JACLYN DUNNE

PRAISE

'Most health books will share amazing advice on how to stay healthy and what to do to keep fit and slim, but *Mind Body Miracle* creates a bridge between all the health theories, tips and tricks around. It takes us deeper into the connection between the physical and spiritual/mental self, allowing miracles to happen. Jaclyn gives practical, helpful and easy to follow information on how to nurture and nourish the mind, only then moving onto the body and capturing the most frequent struggles for us all, such as sugar addiction. The book also provides easy steps to follow to eat better, using the word clean eating in its true form: the consumption of real food. It also provides plans and recipes easy to make at home. The book feels like a conversation had with a knowledgeable friend. I truly enjoyed this read and I will suggest it to all my clients who have to rediscover what it is like to fall in love with their mind and body again.'

**Chantal Di Donato, Author, Speaker,
Health Coach and Founder of Live Lean Health**

'Brilliant and down to earth! Jaclyn Dunne, through the sharing of her own story, is encompassing what medicine is or more rightfully what it should be all about.

You will not put the book down, even if Jaclyn mentions in the beginning that her book doesn't require to be read from cover to cover, I can say you will. She zeros in on the main causes behind inflammation and how our thoughts intrinsically affect our health – the basis of epigenetics, yet explained with the heart of the writer. A must read!'

Christine Marmoy BSc, PT, MCMA Author and Founder of the Detox and Allergy Clinic, London and Spain.

'This book is all about adding value to humanity, adding value to the lives of people who are willing to think into situations and not just about them. People who are willing to change to live! People who want to live in the now and not in the past, who realise that you are what you eat but only to 50%, the other half being – you are what you think.

'It is an inspiring story, a real-life journey by Jaclyn Dunne who has actually walked her talk. She has gone within to not go without and she did it from the inside-out, through action and behaviour; and from the outside-in through attraction.'

Johann Ilgenfritz, Founder and CEO, UK Health Radio Network

RƎTHINK PRESS

First published in Great Britain 2017
by Rethink Press (www.rethinkpress.com)

© Copyright Jaclyn Dunne

CONTENTS

For Mum: I had to lose you to find me

FOREWORD

I thoroughly enjoyed reading *Mind Body Miracle*.

Jaclyn's personal experience with poor health is unfortunately very common with today's modern lifestyle. She was able to successfully navigate her way back to a healthy, positive and fulfilling life experience. The great thing is that Jaclyn has filled her book with valuable and insightful information that will enable you to navigate yourself back to health and happiness. This lovely, informative book gives you a step by step guide to address your wellbeing and lifestyle choices, which will positively affect the physical, mental and emotional aspects of your health.

Oftentimes, it is a lack of awareness of ourselves and our daily choices that create the opportunities to experience poor health. With *Mind Body Miracle* you now have the information to easily empower yourself back to health and happiness.

Thank you, Jaclyn, for such a lovely gift to helping humanity recover its health."

Emma Lane, Naturopath (ND), Functional Medicine Practitioner, Director of Lane Wellness Group – www.lanewellnessgroup.co.uk

INTRODUCTION

The purpose of this book is to provide an easy-to-use tool kit of healthy habits and daily disciplines for anyone who feels that they have lost direction. I have included the strategies and techniques that I use on a daily basis to help my clients bring about the positive changes they so desire. Whether you need focus and clarity to achieve a goal, you want to take the health of your mind and body to the next level, or are seeking strength in adversity, this book will help to support your transformation.

Whatever your goals, *Mind Body Miracle* is a straightforward guide that provides a way of introducing healthy new habits and disciplines into your daily routine for the rest of your life.

Whether you have already begun a journey towards optimum health but would like more direction, or have neglected your health for some time and want to make changes, this book can help.

In two separate, easy-to-follow sections, this book provides clear guidance on how to optimise the health of both your mind and body.

Throughout history, the mind has often been overlooked in discussions on health and wellness. As I detail in the section on the mind, scientific research reveals that the average person has between 50,000 and 70,000 thoughts every day, of which 80% may be negative. Research also states that the sensation of fear stimulates more than 1,400 known physical and chemical responses, activating over 30 different hormones.

In the section on the body, facts and figures backed up by scientific research will motivate you to make positive changes. Here you will find tools to empower you with the knowledge to transform your body into the fully-functioning, healthy 'machine' it was designed to be. Where do you start with this task when you are confronted with a realisation such as that? *Mind, Body Miracle* holds the key.

If you feel as if you are standing at the foot of a mountain wondering how you will ever reach the top, then this book is for you. The book is arranged in two easy-to-follow sections. Each section is designed to encourage and empower you, removing the apprehension that can so often accompany change. You can read it all the way through or dip in and out to find the sections most useful to you at any time.

Each chapter begins with a brief synopsis of how that section can help you, so you can quickly decide what is useful for you.

At the end of every chapter you will find a brief list of action points to help you form new daily habits. It's best to introduce one new healthy habit at a time to make each change sustainable. Although this may sound painstakingly slow, it is far better to cement one positive change than to become overwhelmed and defeated by attempting too many at a time.

If it takes several months to accomplish all the action points, so be it. As the Chinese philosopher Confucius said, it doesn't matter how slowly you go, as long as you do not stop.

PROLOGUE

My mother used to joke that she couldn't go to the bathroom without a little spectator – me. Perhaps it stemmed from my dad leaving us when I was four, which left me clingy and insecure. Mum became my security blanket. I was a sickly child, and if there was a bug going around I caught it. I also had chronic asthma and eczema and was a fussy eater, hardly eating at all on some days. Between the ages of five and eleven, antibiotics were part of my staple diet. That is probably one of the reasons why I went on to be diagnosed with an autoimmune condition at the age of 21.

After struggling through puberty and adolescence, pale, thin and exhausted, at the age of 20 I started to faint regularly. At that time I was working in the City of London as an assistant accountant, and I studied most evenings to become a qualified accountant. I assumed that my fainting episodes were linked to being physically and mentally drained. I explained to my GP that I felt highly emotional, suffered palpitations and fainting spells, and felt chronically fatigued. Initially I was offered anti-depressants, which I refused, and I was then prescribed iron tablets instead.

The fainting episodes continued, becoming more and more frequent. I was now passing out up to three times a week, often on the tube on the way to work. This was both frightening and dangerous, and it involved my boyfriend (now husband) collecting me from a variety of hospitals across London on a weekly basis. After a series of tests, including a bone marrow biopsy, urine tests and multiple blood tests, I was diagnosed with 'pernicious anaemia', or B12 deficiency, as it is now more commonly known.

It was explained that this is not a condition that could be corrected, but only 'managed'. My body had lost the ability to absorb B12, a vitamin crucial for the health of nerves and red blood cells. It is also one of the eight B vitamins that convert food into glucose to provide energy. In order for my body to obtain and utilise B12, it would now need to be injected directly into my bloodstream every month for the foreseeable future. At the time I thought this was a small price to pay for feeling better and, with blind faith, I asked few questions.

By the time I was 25, I was struggling with life. I had qualified as an accountant; I was planning my wedding; and working exceptionally long hours for a logistics company in East London. The pernicious anaemia was described by my consultant haematologist as 'under control'. I was now having B12 injections every three months and the final month before an injection was an arduous time.

My mum and stepfather had now moved to Peterborough, which was two hours' drive away. Not only did I miss them terribly, but my mum had started to get frequent chest infections. She was forced into early retirement and was put on steroids, at just 54. Chest infections turned into pneumonia, which left scarring on her lungs, and she was also struggling to get through a month without a hospital stay. My mum had always been fiercely independent, and now my step-dad was her carer. I spent the next ten years in a state of acute anxiety. I was terrified that Mum wouldn't be able to come to my wedding after one particularly frightening incident that resulted in her going into respiratory arrest. When I became pregnant with my first daughter (and then my second) I was afraid that Mum would never get to hold them. My own illness was also increasingly worrying, particularly during my two pregnancies. I didn't have enough B12 for myself, let alone for a baby growing inside me. This led me to have three iron infusions and two blood transfusions during both of my pregnancies. I was so completely drained that I could hardly function. I was signed off work when I was six weeks' pregnant with my first child, but the second time around I managed to work part-time up until 38 weeks.

I spent as much time as I could visiting my mum, particularly now that I only worked for part of each week. I used my days off to be with her, as she loved to spend time with my babies and me. However, Mum's diagnosis was now Chronic Obstructive Pulmonary Disease (COPD), which meant that it was only a matter of time before she became oxygen-dependent, and therefore housebound.

In January 2013, as I turned 35, my mum was placed in palliative care. Her lungs and body were ravaged from 10 years of high-dose steroids, she was oxygen-dependent, and, at only 64 she had had enough. On 28th January, after my sister and I spent an entire day sitting holding Mum's hand, her suffering ended. I was devastated beyond words.

While I planned Mum's funeral, wrote a eulogy and plodded on with my parental duties as best I could, I went on to autopilot. Then, just five days after my mother passed away, I received the news that my biological father had just hours to live, following a massive stroke. My dad had not been a huge part of my life after having left when I was four, and I made the decision that I couldn't watch another parent die in that same week. So. I never got to see my father before the news came, a few hours later, that he had passed away. Looking back, I now realise that I was raw and numb from the loss of my beloved mother, I was so dazed and shocked that I struggled to eat or sleep, and felt an enormous sense of loneliness at that time.

I turned to my sister Jo, the only person who could know what I was feeling. Although we didn't live close to each other, we spoke daily on the phone, clinging to each other's voice for comfort. One evening, my mum had been gone for six weeks when, after a phone call with my sister, I sat in uncontrollable sobs as a conversation with my mum shortly before she died came back to me: *'Jac, when I go, you can cry for a little but not for long, and certainly not forever. You have your own family to look after now and I'll be watching as you make me proud.'*

In that moment, sitting on the sofa without her, I knew that I had some huge changes to make.

HEALING

I had begun the process of evaluating my life. My mother's death had taught me that we only have a limited time to *live*. I was doing a job that I didn't enjoy, neglecting my own health and wallowing in my own misery. I was just existing, and I needed to *live* while I was alive, by following my dreams and my passions.

Since losing her grandmother, my eldest daughter had needed counselling. They were particularly close, and at only four years old my daughter was struggling to make sense of the situation. I saw a huge change in her behaviour since she gained the support to work through her emotions. The positive impact that counselling had on my child made me feel that my job as an accountant was insignificant. My mum used to tell me and my sister that we should try to leave the world a little better than we found it. I then decided that I wanted to make a difference, so I applied for a three-year counselling course.

When I arrived for the interview I was told that the first year of the course was hypnotherapy. I asked the interviewer if it was absolutely necessary to do a year of hypnotherapy, since I was adamant that I wanted to focus on counselling. He explained that hypnotherapy is a useful tool for counsellors, so the first year was mandatory. I was accepted on the course and decided to give it a go.

The course provided the perfect distraction from my grief, and although I was still subject to tearful outbursts, I focused on my mum's words. I also started to read self-development books and introduce a new set of daily disciplines into my routine, including affirmations, meditations and gratitude lists. These new

7

daily habits helped to keep my mind focused and my thoughts positive.

My course was teaching me the power of the subconscious mind, and my new daily habits served as a reminder. Despite my earlier reservations, I was captivated by hypnotherapy and its many uses. Six months into my diploma we covered 'hypnotherapy for weight management', and I sat in complete awe of how powerful a tool this was. Not only could it change lives, but potentially save lives too.

I rushed home to my husband, telling him that I wanted to become a hypnotherapist specialising in weight. James, who is often the voice of reason, pointed out that it would be far better to have some knowledge of nutrition if I was helping people to manage their weight. I immediately enrolled on a nutrition course to run alongside my diploma in hypnotherapy and counselling. My life became a whirlwind of studying and essay writing. As luck would have it, I was also informed that I was surplus to requirements in my accountancy job. I took this as a sign from my mum and the universe that I was now on the right path.

Amid all the studying and parenting I truly neglected my health. I was certainly tired, but who wouldn't be with that workload, two children and a house to run? However, a sudden fainting episode, followed by a letter from the hospital (stating that I had missed two haematology appointments) served as the reminder that I so badly needed.

When I eventually saw my consultant, he was far from impressed that I had not had a B12 injection for 18 months, and had failed to attend my assessments for a year. He explained that I had jeopardised my health and risked damage to my nervous system through failing to have an injection. I told him that I had suffered a double loss and was busy studying, but he asserted that my health had not been my priority. I disagreed, as my health had become a huge priority since I started to study nutrition and hypnotherapy. I was fuelling my body with what it needed in terms of vitamins and minerals, and had adopted a positive and focused mind-set. He reminded me that my body could no longer absorb B12, regardless of how I ate, which is why I needed the injection. I promised him that I would see my GP for a B12 injection in the next week, as my haemoglobin levels were dropping. Little did I know that this was to be the last B12 injection that I ever needed.

After starting to read about the vast subject of nutrition, and having been diagnosed with B12 deficiency, which is an autoimmune disease, I became fascinated by autoimmune conditions, how they manifest and how they are treated.

An autoimmune disease occurs when your immune system, which is your line of defence against disease, attacks healthy cells in the belief that they are foreign invaders. There is an ever-growing list of diseases categorised as 'autoimmune', from diabetes to rheumatoid arthritis, Crohn's disease, psoriasis, and lupus. Autoimmune disease is even linked to many types of cancer. As I was learning from my own experiences, conventional medicine advises that there is no cure for autoimmune conditions, only management. Management comes in the form of lifelong medication, which can actually involve *suppressing* the immune system, the body's defence against disease. Furthermore, most medications come with a long list of unwelcome side effects, such as fatigue, weight gain and depression, often making further medication necessary. Doing my own research made me feel disheartened with the medical profession. I felt disappointed because much of what I researched myself had never been explained to me. I had no idea that pernicious anaemia was even classed as an autoimmune condition, meaning that my immune system was under attack. In the ten years since my diagnosis no-one in the medical profession had spoken to me about how to strengthen my immune system, nor advised me about my diet and lifestyle, and I certainly did not feel as though the B12 injections were coming close to treating the root cause of the deficiency.

From my nutrition studies, I understood that B12 was absorbed in a part of the small intestines called the ileum. During digestion stomach acid assists in releasing B12 from protein in foods. Once released, B12 combines with a digestive enzyme called 'intrinsic factor' before it is absorbed into the bloodstream. I desperately wanted to understand why this process had stopped taking place in my body. Craving a deeper understanding of why I was no longer absorbing an essential vitamin, I continued my studies into autoimmune disease and came across Dr Alessio Fasano, a world-renowned gastroenterologist, research scientist and expert on 'intestinal permeability and its connection to autoimmune disorders'. Dr Fasano stated that there is a strong body of evidence highlighting intestinal permeability (also known as 'leaky gut syndrome') as a major cause of autoimmune issues.

Having recently completed a unit on my nutrition course covering 'gut microbiome and the importance of gut health', I was aware that the digestive system houses 80% of our immune system. A light bulb moment!

B12 is absorbed in the gut, so you cannot have a healthy immune system without a healthy gut, because the immune system resides in the gut. Furthermore, research by a world leader in this field had shown undeniable links between a 'leaking' gut and autoimmune disorders, which my condition was classified as being.

I strongly suspected that the root cause of my B12 deficiency was intestinal permeability. My gut lining had worn away and it was allowing much of what was passing through my intestines to enter my bloodstream. These particles are then recognised by the immune system as foreign invaders worthy of attack. Upon further research I discovered that many doctors practising functional medicine attributed the malabsorption of vital minerals and nutrients (such as B12, zinc, magnesium and iron), to poor gut health). So, how had my gut become so unhealthy that it had possibly started to leak, triggering an autoimmune response?

The average length of the small intestine is 3–5 metres. It assists in digestion, as well as acting as a barrier to keep harmful gut contents out of the bloodstream. There are three main reasons why the junctions between the intestinal cells get wider, causing matter passing through the gut to escape: an over-processed diet, chronic stress, and toxic overload, in particular alcohol and medication. Although I had never had a particularly processed diet, I had suffered several periods of chronic stress, as well as a toxic onslaught from antibiotics as a child. Antibiotics are prescribed to kill bacterial infections. Unfortunately they kill both the good and the bad bacteria in our guts. If we are not doing enough to replace the friendly bacteria in our intestines, we are jeopardising our immune systems and our overall health. I could finally connect the dots of my B12 deficiency and begin the process of healing my gut.

By following a simple three-step approach (see the Heal Your Gut chapter of this book), as well as ensuring that I ate well, reduced my levels of stress and also toxins, I have not needed a B12 injection for several years now.

I have become so enthused by holistic living that I am continuing my studies with the CHEK institute to become a holistic lifestyle coach, having completed Level 1 in 2015. I'm also continuing my professional development by attending regular courses and workshops in this area.

My experience has made me passionate about empowering others with the tools that I wish I had been given when conventional medicine failed me during my struggle with an autoimmune condition, and when my life skills weren't enough for me to cope with the turbulence of life.

My story isn't special – we all go through difficult times. It's not the experience that defines us; it's the way that we handle it.

PROLOGUE

Being broken gives you the opportunity to build yourself again, stronger than ever. In my experience, I had to go through the worst time of my life to arrive at the best. I now have a new career, new outlook, mind-set and passion. This is my legacy to my mum – and the irony is not lost in that I had to lose her in order to find *me*.

MIND

DAILY AFFIRMATIONS

*'The secret of your success is found in
your daily routine.'*
JOHN C. MAXWELL

This chapter will help if you:

- Want to be able to self-motivate

- Have little self-belief and lack confidence

- Need focus and clarity to achieve a goal

Positive affirmations are short, powerful statements of support and encouragement composed to inspire, energize and motivate both your conscious and subconscious mind.

Louise Hay, the author, motivational speaker and founder of the self-help movement describes affirmations as, 'a beginning point on the path to change.'

You are already performing affirmations on a daily basis – we all are. But are they positive? That is highly unlikely, since we are our own worst critics; guilty of negative self-talk and an internal dialogue that limits our self-belief. The fact is that we would never talk to others the way that we talk to ourselves with our automatic negative thoughts or ANT, as experts refer to it as. For example, would you walk up to a school mum in the playground, as her child went into school feeling unsettled and tearful, and tell them what a terrible parent they are? It's extremely unlikely – but your internal dialogue with yourself on such a morning might be 'I am such a bad mum.' Right?

As another example, a friend is flicking through a magazine and sighs longingly at the slender models. Do you say to your friend 'You are much too fat and really should start that diet you keep banging on about?' That's even more unlikely – but you may tell yourself that.

Recent research suggests that humans have between 50,000 and 70,000 thoughts a day, with as much as 80% of them being negative. This means that most of the time we are affirming our shortcomings and our failures to ourselves.

Just imagine if you could reset your thoughts and words into positive patterns that, in turn, bring about positive change. Well you can, by writing your own positive affirmations and repeating them daily.

There are many benefits to making positive affirmations part of your daily routine.

Firstly, by ensuring that you are including positive language in your daily self-talk you will start to become more aware of your inner dialogue and thought process. Slowly but surely, negative language becomes less frequent as positivity becomes more habitual.

Additionally, by incorporating affirmations into your daily

routine you can keep your goals in clear focus, as you remind yourself of them each time you speak your affirmations aloud.

I always give my hypnotherapy clients an affirmation to work into their daily routine, in order to reaffirm the messages and suggestions that we have planted in the subconscious mind during the hypnotherapy session. The subconscious mind is where we store all our learned habits and behaviours that become automated over time. However, with continual reminders in the form of daily affirmations, these habits can be reprogrammed if you so wish.

In my opinion, one of the most satisfying reasons to say daily affirmations is that positivity is even more contagious than the common cold.

I personally find it impossible to stay feeling down or not return a smile when I am around someone who is upbeat. However, negativity can be just as infectious, and if you are with people who are constantly negative it can be immensely difficult to remain in a positive mood. Surround yourself with people who lift your energy, or vibration , and limit your time around those that don't. By identifying your 'positive posse' you will find it much easier to re-programme positivity in your mind. Also, make a decision to be the light-giver, the patron saint of smiling, the positivity spreader, and you will be amazed at who you attract into your tribe when you lift your vibration higher. If you are going to spread anything contagious, it is far better for it to be the feeling of positivity!

According to a study carried out by LD Kubzansky et al in 2007 at Harvard School of Public Health, optimistic people experience biological benefits. The study revealed that people with a more positive outlook on life were less likely to experience high cholesterol, high blood pressure and even obesity. The most optimistic individuals were 50% less likely to experience a cardiovascular episode, such as a heart attack or stroke, compared to their less optimistic peers.

Affirmations are simple to write but they must be worded in a specific way in order to instil self-belief and bring to life your strengths and skills. Although there are already many excellent affirmations in books and online, it is far better to write your own. When I give my clients affirmations, I generally encourage them to re-word them as if they had written them.

When writing your own affirmations you will naturally use the language and tone that you are accustomed to in everyday life. This makes the affirmation far more acceptable and recognisable to the subconscious mind, and leaves little room for hesitancy and doubt.

The most important rule to remember when creating an affirmation is that it needs to be written in the present tense, as if you have already achieved the goal. For example, if your goal is being a dress size 10 by the summer of 2017, you would write,

'It is June 2017, and I feel fabulous in my size 10 dress.'

This affirmation has all the ingredients to be successfully accepted and recognised by the subconscious mind. Firstly, it has a time scale, secondly, it has a specific goal and finally, it is written in the present tense. The subconscious does not respond well to vague instructions, so by giving a date and a dress size, you are making the goal specific and adding a deadline, which is easy for the subconscious mind to process and act upon. Also, the subconscious mind only understands the here and now. If the affirmation was written, ' I want to feel fabulous in my size 10 dress by June 2017,' what the subconscious mind hears is 'want' and it will respond with ways to make you 'want' to feel fabulous, which of course is what you already desire on a conscious level. The end result will not result in any change, as your 'want' will simply get stronger and your goal will feel further out of reach.

To understand fully the best ways to structure your affirmations for maximum impact and results, let's take a look at some ill-considered versions of the previous example; **'I don't want to be fat anymore'**

This example is not setting a goal, as it is focusing on what you no longer want. It is generally accepted amongst hypnotherapists that the subconscious mind is not very good at processing negatives such as 'don't', 'can't' and 'won't'. A book I would highly recommend that explains this concept well is *Drop The Pink Elephant* by Bill McFarlan. If I said to you, 'Don't think of a pink elephant,' it is highly likely that you now have a vivid image of a pink elephant in your mind. This is a simple example of the subconscious mind not processing negatives. This is useful information to remember when you are communicating with children. 'Don't run' compared to 'walk carefully' will bring about a different reaction and outcome, even though we perceive them as having the same meaning.

'I'm going to try to be a size 10 by June 2017' This phrase will not have the desired effect on the subconscious mind for the same reason as using the word 'want'. The subconscious mind will focus on what you are 'trying' to do and just keep you 'trying'. Your actions will echo the strength of your request, and this request has an undertone of failure. Avoid using phrases such as 'I want,' 'I will try', and 'I will attempt'.

'I will be a size 10 by June 2017' This affirmation is referring to the future, rather than the present, so is not definitive enough. It is also missing the emotional language. In our perfect example, we used the words 'I feel fabulous', combining the instruction with an emotional reaction, which will ignite feelings of motivation.

'I am a size 10' Although this affirmation is specific, to the point and in the present tense, it does not give a timescale. An affirmation without a timescale is too vague for the subconscious to act upon, and it does not add any urgency. Once again, there is no emotive language to make you *feel* the affirmation as well as *hear* it. Ideally, saying your affirmation aloud will trigger several emotions, such as excitement, inspiration, motivation and happiness.

When I first started to do affirmations I felt a bit of a fraud. There I was, standing in front of the mirror saying out loud how happy and healthy I felt, while a little voice deep inside was saying, 'who are you trying to kid with this woo-woo nonsense?' The best piece of advice that I can give when negativity is creeping into your mind is something that my mum used to tell my sister and me, 'Fake it till you make it.'

Say your affirmations aloud daily and eventually you will silence your biggest critic – *you*.

Since your affirmations are a new habit to include in your daily routine, it can be easy to forget to do them. The best way I have found to do affirmations is to anchor them to an existing daily habit that you are unlikely to forget. In my world that is cleaning my teeth, as I clean my teeth twice a day, without fail. In the bathroom I have hung four small frames next to my toothbrush, and each heart-shaped frame contains a written affirmation. These serve as a reminder to say the affirmations when I brush my teeth. I now find it really difficult to perform teeth brushing without saying my affirmations immediately afterwards because I have created a new habit – and you can too.

Finally, you can change or update your affirmations whenever you want to. Obviously the most sensible time would be once you have achieved a goal. I find that four affirmations said twice daily are more than manageable. However, there are no rules as to how many affirmations to use at once, or how many times a day to say them, as long as you are able to incorporate them into your daily routine.

By writing affirmations in your own words, in the present tense, with a positive outcome, giving a deadline and saying them aloud at least twice a day; you are implementing a positive daily discipline. This will help to build your self-belief and self-worth, as well as giving you focus, clarity and motivation while working towards any goal.

ACTION POINTS

- Write three positive affirmations using your own words, with a positive tone and in the present tense. Give your affirmations a timescale by including a deadline, and remember to use 'feeling' words.

- Decide which daily habit you will anchor your affirmations to, to ensure they will be said at least once a day without fail.

- Place the affirmations where you will see them everyday, and ideally close to where you perform your 'anchor' habit.

- Recite them daily, loud and proud, with as much emotion as you can muster and simply wait for the magic to happen.

AN ATTITUDE OF GRATITUDE

*'Trade your expectation for appreciation and the
world changes instantly.'*
TONY ROBBINS

This chapter will help if you:

- Are suffering from depression

- Need a tool kit to wash away anger, aggression
  and apathy

- Want to reduce your negative mind-set and raise
  your vibration

My mother always told me to remember my Ps and Qs, and
drummed the message home to instil good manners. She was
possibly not aware of the huge benefits of cultivating gratitude
as a daily habit.

When I speak to my clients about using 'daily gratitude tools',
they generally question that something so simple could bring
about such huge shifts.

In this chapter we will look at the scientifically proven
benefits of cultivating an 'attitude of gratitude', the effortless

routines of acknowledgment that can transform physical and mental well-being, and the reasons why you need to replace your vision board with a gratitude board instead!

Robert A. Emmons, the psychologist, leading gratitude researcher and author of *Gratitude Works* and *The Psychology of Gratitude* has conducted many studies on the link between gratitude and well-being. His findings conclude that practicing daily gratitude effectively increases happiness and reduces depression. When I work with clients who are suffering from depression, they often feel offended by the suggestion that gratitude may assist them. I can't say that I blame them. In dark times, if someone had told me to look on the bright side I would have also taken offence. Depressed clients tell me that they have nothing to be thankful for. In response to this, I share one of my favourites quotes by the poet and novelist, Charles Bukowski,

> *'There is a light somewhere, it may not be much light, but it beats the darkness'.*

When we look for things to be thankful for (however small), we begin to focus more on the positives in our lives. An added bonus is that this way of thinking actually changes the brain chemistry that is the hallmark of depression. Research by Dr Joshua Brown from Indiana University in 2015 found that the brain almost has a 'gratitude muscle' and the more that gratitude is practised, the more the brain adapts to this mind-set.

Further studies by Nathan Dewall et al in 2012, from the

University of Kentucky showed that those who ranked higher on gratitude scales were less likely to retaliate against others, even when they were shown aggression and negativity, and instead they showed sensitivity and empathy.

However, it is not just psychological health that can be improved by showing gratitude; physical health can improve too. Paul Mills, US Professor of Family Medicine and Public Health at the San Diego School of Medicine, University of California, conducted studies in 2015 that looked at the role of gratitude on heart health. In one of his findings participants who kept a daily journal of three things that they were grateful for had reduced levels of inflammation and a better heart rhythm than those that did not have this 'gratitude' habit.

Additionally, grateful people are able to appreciate and celebrate other people's accomplishments. So many of us are guilty of making social comparisons, whether we care to admit to it or not – cars, houses, jobs, holidays, children, salaries, handbags, shoes – the comparing and measuring can be endless. This mind-set is toxic, leads to feelings of resentment and is a major contributing factor in reducing one's self-esteem. Grateful people are able to appreciate others' accomplishments without feeling bitter or jealous. Imagine the freedom if you released the unnecessary pressure to 'keep up with the neighbours'. It is time we accepted that happiness is not linked to financial wealth and material possessions. According to social progress polls, the countries with the highest standard of financial living are not necessarily the happiest.

It was exactly one year after losing my mum that I started to cultivate a daily gratitude habit. You may think that a strange time to start counting my blessings, but on the first anniversary of my mother's death her words rang in my ears. She had specifically asked me to not spend the rest of my life in mourning. I was still struggling emotionally, but as I laid flowers on her grave I vowed to be thankful for the times we had together, to smile at the memories and to focus on the blessings in my life instead of what I was lacking.

That night I tucked my children into bed with immense gratitude that I had two beautiful, healthy girls, and from that day on I began my daily gratitude habits. It wasn't until months later that I read a research paper on positive psychology, which stated that negative life events did not necessarily lower a person's level of happiness in the long-term if they practised gratitude. The article concluded that a pre-event level of happiness usually returns within two years. I know from my own painful experience that directly after the loss of a loved one you feel as though life will never be the same again. This is absolutely true, since life will not be the same without my mum, but that does not mean that I cannot be happy without her. I can, and I will. Gratitude contributes hugely to one's resilience. Recognise all that you have to be thankful for, even in the worst of times.

> 'Count your blessings, not your crosses,
> Count your gains, not your losses.
> Count your joys instead of your woes,

Count your friends, instead of your foes.
Count your smiles instead of your tears,
Count your courage instead of your fears.
Count your health, not your wealth
Love your neighbour as much as yourself
IRISH BLESSING

In the best-selling book and film, *The Secret*, Rhonda Byrne suggests how to use the Law of Attraction. The principles of *The Secret* are claimed to be based on quantum physics, supporting the idea that like attracts like and what you put out you will attract back to yourself. Before *The Secret* many had not heard of this universal law. However, Napoleon Hill wrote the first bestseller on the subject of the Law of Attraction, called *Think and Grow Rich* back in 1937. Prior to this, there were many religious teachings in alignment with the Law of Attraction. The Hindu concept of Karma states,

'Whatsoever a man soweth,
that shall he also reap.'

An all-time favourite quote of mine is from Buddha,

'All that we are is the result of what we
have thought. The mind is everything.
What we think we become.'

There has also been much research into the science behind the Law of Attraction and whether it can be proven. However, I see this universal law much more as a spiritual practice than a scientific theory.

One thing I would like to challenge which features in the Law of Attraction is the use of 'vision boards'. A vision or dream board is a visual representation of the things that you would like to have and achieve in your life. I admit that my children and I have been known to make vision boards, and would use them to display pictures of the things we wanted: a bigger house, faster car, pet dog (in the case of my children), award at school, or promotion at work. However, a good friend whom I classed as my spiritual teacher questioned my use of vision boards. She pointed out that if the Law of Attraction states that you get back what you put out, vision boards will actually keep you in a place of 'lack'. That was a moment of realisation. A vision board is showing all the things that you *want* so you stay *wanting* because like attracts like. It also serves as a visual reminder of all the things that you don't have, which can create feelings of resentment and low self-worth. She suggested that a gratitude board is far more beneficial as a way of acknowledging the things you are most grateful for. It not only puts your life into a positive perspective, it will attract more of the same – things to be grateful for. The best-selling author, Lewis Howes, writes in his book *The School of Greatness*, 'If you concentrate on what you have, you'll always have more. If you concentrate on what you don't have, you'll never have enough.'

My children and I have since swapped our yearly vision

boards for gratitude boards, which I frequently stare at and smile with an overwhelming feeling of love and appreciation.

For gratitude to become a state of mind, it must first become a way of life. This is far easier than you might think, as it simply means carving out a little time in your day to implement gratitude habits and to express thanks for all the people and things in your life. This does not mean that you have no room for negative thoughts or feelings, as that would be difficult and unnatural. It is also detrimental to your health to deny or disguise feelings of pain and discomfort. Daily gratitude habits are to search for and recognise points of light, even in darkness.

Here are my top five ways to cultivate a daily attitude of gratitude:

1. Write a gratitude list

Each morning write a short list of three new things that you are grateful for. It is important that you think of *new* things, as this ensures that your gratitude remains fresh. This is part of my morning routine with my children. From the ages of four and seven they started to make a written list of three things they are grateful for each day. Not only does this serve as a positive start to the day, but is also entertaining and enlightening to hear what your children are grateful for. My youngest daughter is a foodie and often grateful for the dinner she was served the previous evening. My eldest daughter is often grateful for people's actions and kind words. We keep our daily gratitude lists in a journal and they are a wonderful keepsake.

2. Keep a gratitude journal

As well as noting down three new points of gratitude each morning for the day ahead, I also make a note of three things that I am grateful for at the end of the day. This means that my gratitude list has six points in total each day. According to a 2011 study by psychology professor, Nancy Digdon, entitled 'Gratitude Interventions on Sleep Quality' and published in *Applied Psychology Health and Well-Being,* spending a few minutes noting down grateful sentiments before bed will help you to sleep better and for longer.

3. Look back and acknowledge

At the end of each week, in your gratitude journal, make a note of things you have accomplished and feel proud of. We are often advised that there is no point in looking back, but it is beneficial to be reminded just how far you have come. This will also help in building your self-esteem and confidence.

4. Give thanks to others

At the end of each day, use your gratitude journal to make a note of people who have inspired, helped or supported you, and remember to thank them. You have the power to lift someone higher just by using two little words – 'thank you'.

5. Make a gratitude board

Put together a collage of all the things that you are grateful for in your life. I have used an app on my phone to make a visual reminder of all that I am proud of. This can include a warm home, a loving heart, healthy children, a healthy body, love, and security. Simply ask yourself the question, 'What am I grateful for?' and find a picture to symbolise this. It doesn't matter how small things seem, as Robert Braulte wrote:

> 'Enjoy the little things, for one day you may look
> back and realise they were the big things.'

I view my gratitude collage at least five times a day, as it is saved to my mobile phone, but you could also make it into a screen saver on your computer or a picture for a frame.

Although these five points may seem a lot to remember, with practice they will become as automatic and habitual as brushing your teeth. The multitude of benefits felt by implementing daily gratitude habits far outweigh the little time that they take to cultivate. Gratitude is far more than good manners – it is one of the most healing emotions that we can feel. Remind yourself daily of all that you have to be grateful for and enjoy the positive changes that this practice brings to your mind-set, your health and your relationships.

ACTION POINTS

- Keep a daily gratitude journal to give thanks for all you have.

- Write in the journal before bed to improve sleep, or make a mental note of the positives in your day as you drift off.

- Every day, thank someone who has helped or inspired you.

- Take time to acknowledge your own accomplishments. Praise yourself and become your new best friend instead of your worst enemy and biggest critic.

MEDITATIONS AND VISUALISATIONS

*'A calm mind is the ultimate weapon
against your challenges'*
BRYANT MCGILL

This chapter will help if you:

- Have a restless mind and struggle to gain focus
  and clarity

- Would like to increase your happiness, health and
  energy by spending ten minutes a day relaxing

- Want more confidence and self-belief to reach
  your goals.

Our modern world is busy, chaotic and noisy, and as a result our minds have become the same. Technology provides us with 24-hour stimulation, making it hard to find a place of peace and quiet, even when we desperately want to. Furthermore, the meteoric rise of social media sites for both business and pleasure has kept us busy connecting to everyone – apart from ourselves. This is a huge irony of modern times. As we become more and more busy, building our external profile and seeking inspiration for growth, the inspiration that we seek is actually within, if we would only be silent and listen.

Meditation is a mind-body practice rapidly on the rise in the West, yet still only 8% of the US regularly practise it and there are no known stats for the UK. Perhaps this is because many believe that meditation is only for spiritual bohemians and Buddhists, or maybe they are simply unaware of the full extent of proven benefits.

Meditation is the practice of turning your attention to a single point of reference. It can involve focusing on the breath, on bodily sensations, or on a word or phrase, known as a 'mantra'. Quite simply, meditation is silencing any distracting thoughts and tuning into your inner world to de-clutter your mind and gain perspective.

There are over 3,000 scientific studies on the benefits of meditation. Some of these studies indicate that meditating for just 20 minutes per day for a few weeks is enough to experience such benefits as:

- Reduced anxiety and depression
- Increased self-esteem
- Increased focus
- ADHD management
- Increased immunity
- Reduced blood pressure
- Reduced inflammation
- Improved cognitive health

In January 2014, *Journal of the American Medical Association* (JAMA) published a study led by Dr.Madhav Goyal at the John Hopkins University stating meditation to be as effective in the treatment of depression as antidepressant drugs.

Three studies, carried out by Alberto Chiesa M.D of the Institute of Psychiatry at the University of Bologna, published in the *Journal of Alternative and Complementary Medicine*, suggested that meditation could help to reduce alcohol and substance abuse.

A study of adults with attention deficit hyperactivity disorder (ADHD), published in the *Clinical Neurophysiology* Journal (see details on References page), documented how a group submitted to Mindfulness-based Cognitive Therapy (MBCT) demonstrated reduced hyperactivity and reduced impulsivity, contributing to an overall improvement in symptoms.

It is apparent from existing medical research that meditation is a powerful healing tool, and one that is hugely underestimated.

When I first started to use meditation as a daily discipline, I had little idea of what I was doing. I read up on the different types of meditation practice, such as Vipassana, which means 'insight', and Anapanasati, which focuses on breath. I was concerned that I would not have the correct technique. Did I need to learn a mantra or burn some incense? Did I need to sit in a certain position for a given length of time,? I decided that for me, the best way to begin meditating was not to over-think it. It was Zig Ziglar who said,

> *'You don't have to be great to start, but you
> do have to start to be great.'*

BEGINNERS GUIDE TO MEDITATION: SEVEN SMALL STEPS TO CALMNESS

Step 1 – Make a commitment

Like all the other healthy habits and daily disciplines in this book, meditation is easy to do and provides huge benefits when one is consistent. There is little point in starting with a 'give it a go' attitude. The cumulative effect is necessary to reap the rewards. Commit to at least a month of daily meditation practice before deciding whether or not it is helping you. You will enjoy the daily relaxation and 'me time' if nothing else.

Step 2 – Start small

I started small, investing just three minutes each day into my practice. As I grew used to this discipline, I slowly and gradually increased the time. Set a timer with a gentle alarm to alert you when your minutes have expired. This is something that you will come to rely on as your practice becomes longer and deeper.

Step 3 – Develop a routine

I made sure that I meditated at the same time every day so that it quickly became a routine daily discipline. Research has shown that it is much easier to create a new daily habit when it is done at the same time each day. I chose the morning as it fitted into my schedule and I could commit to it. There is probably not a 'best' time to meditate, although first thing in the morning is a wonderful start to the day and last thing at night can aid sleep.

Step 4 – Make Yourself Comfortable

I started my practice by sitting up straight, cross-legged on the floor, with my hands resting on my knees. If sitting cross-legged on the floor is not possible or comfortable, simply sit on a chair with your arms and legs unfolded. As long as you can sit somewhere comfortable and quiet, you can begin.

Step 5 – Do a Body Scan

Before relaxing the mind, you must first relax the body. Close your eyes and bring your awareness to each part of your body. Starting at the top of the head and working down, notice any tension that you are holding and release it, allowing yourself to feel supported yet relaxed.

Step 6 – Focus on your Breathing

Once you are comfortable and settled, keep your eyes closed and bring your attention to your breathing. Continue to breathe at a comfortable pace and concentrate on each breath you take, as it comes in through your nose and fills your lungs. It may help you to count each breath, breathing in on one and out on two, continuing this up until the number ten and then returning to one again.

Step 7 – Train your mind to focus

It is an absolute certainty that your mind will drift and wander, which is not a problem. Many friends and clients tell me that they are 'no good' at meditation because their mind keeps wandering.

This is perfectly normal, as our brains continuously produce thoughts, and this process cannot be turned off. In fact, a wandering mind is necessary for meditation to have the desired effect. Just as it would be difficult to teach a dog to sit if it was already sitting, it would be difficult to train your mind to focus if it was not wandering.

Meditation is not about completely clearing your mind, as this would be a virtually impossible task. It is about training yourself to refocus in an effort to quiet a busy head. When you are aware that your mind has drifted, bring your attention back to your breathing and begin counting again, breathing in on number one and out on number two, continuing to ten and repeating.

With regular practice and patience these nourishing, focused states of mind can deepen into profoundly peaceful and energised states of mind. Regular meditation practice is taking the time to become acquainted with yourself and your inner thoughts. It is 'time out' that we rarely have in this frantic world, and this time will reward you with a balanced and stable mind. If you are new to meditation you may find it useful to download a guided meditation app to your computer or phone. Many of these apps are free and user-friendly, particularly for meditation novices. I recommend the *Headspace* app, which gives a series of free ten-minute guided meditations, ideal for newcomers to meditation. There are also many meditation CDs that range from soothing music and mantras to guided breathing and visualisation techniques.

You may decide that you would like to join a meditation group for assistance and guidance. This is also a great way to meet like-minded people who are likely to be on a similar journey of mindfulness and spiritual consciousness. A few months after implementing meditation as a daily discipline, I joined a six-week meditation course at a local Buddhist Centre. This not only introduced me to the history and uses of meditation, but also taught chants, mantras and visualisations. The weeks that I spent meditating at the Buddhist Centre were both calming and enlightening and instigated a journey of spiritual insight and self-awareness. Classes and courses are often available at yoga studios, as yoga is also a meditative exercise. If you want to take your practice further and become part of a meditation group, research what is available locally and decide what resonates with you.

According to the universal law of cause and effect, every action has a reaction. It is not possible to practice regular meditation without also feeling the benefits. These may not be obvious initially, but slowly and gradually the seeds that you sow in your subconscious mind during meditation will come to fruition. Have patience and be gentle with yourself, as the rewards, which may not always be obvious, will most certainly appear. Aside from the health benefits considered earlier in this chapter, you will also see progress through your ability to relax and find emotional calmness, freeing yourself from stresses that once concerned you. You will begin to notice that you are fully present and focused in the here and now, as opposed to having a busy and wandering mind unable to concentrate or retain information. When our mind becomes overloaded with information we often lose clarity and focus. The irony of meditation is that the quieter you become, the more you hear. The late, great philosopher Wayne Dyer summed up meditation when he said,

> *'You cannot always control what goes on outside,*
> *but you can always control what goes on inside.'*

THE POWER OF VISUALISATIONS

Visualisations are the meditative practice of imagining the best possible outcome in a scenario – day-dreaming with a positive purpose. There is much scientific research into the effectiveness of positive visualisations and their incredible benefits.

Visualisation is also known as Mental Imagery, or Visual Mental Rehearsal (VMR), and is a technique proven to be extraordinarily successful in producing a specific outcome. As I explain in the chapter entitled The Power Of The Subconscious Mind, our mind plays a vital role in the creation of our experiences. Research in this field has shown that the brain cannot differentiate between imagining and doing, therefore visualising a successful outcome conditions both the mind and the body to achieve that result.

Many sports and business professionals use this technique of succeeding in their mind to ensure that they do so in reality.

- The Hollywood actor Jim Carrey used to visualise himself as 'the greatest actor in the world' before becoming a star.

- The boxing legend Muhammad Ali spoke about seeing himself as being victorious before a fight.
- Oprah Winfrey has spoken at length on the power of intention and visualisation playing a huge part in her successful career.
- The actor and musician Will Smith has spoken of being an A-list Hollywood superstar in his mind, long before he actually was.
- Athlete, Jessica Ennis-Hill revealed visualisations as her mental training tactic prior to the 2012 London Olympic Games.

These highly successful people and many others have mastered the technique of positive visualisations and credit it as a success tactic.

Australian Psychologist Alan Richardson conducted an experiment with three groups of basketball players. He instructed the first group to practise free throws for 20 minutes daily, while the second group would only visualise themselves making throws and the third group would not practise at all. The results provide astounding evidence for the power of visualisation. The group that only visualised were almost as good as the group who actually practised. Dr David Hamilton PhD has also documented a wealth of evidence that visualisation has been successful in improving health and wellbeing. Having written several books about quantum physics and the mind body connection, he says,

> 'The brain doesn't distinguish real from imaginary.
> As we imagine something, to the brain, what we
> imagine is actually happening. I've shared scientific
> evidence of how people have altered physical
> strength through visualisation, how visualisation
> can help weight loss, as well as how visualisation is
> used to help people heal from illness.'

Visualisation is a simple practice and can be combined with daily meditation. I often use this technique after my ten minutes of morning meditation. I remain still and silent and visualise exactly how I would like my day to go, especially if I have something particularly important planned. I also visualise positive outcomes for my family and even my clients.

SEVEN SIMPLE STEPS TO CREATE VISUALISATIONS

Step 1. Use the seven steps to calmness to create the perfect headspace for powerful visualisations.

Step 2. Start your visualisation by imagining the environment in as clear, concise and detailed a way as possible.

Step 3. Engage all of the senses as you create the scene. What can you see? How does it smell? What can you hear? Is there something to touch or taste?

Step 4. The more vivid you can imagine the scene, the more your brain will accept it as fact, so spend time building a strong image.

Step 5. Imagine the scene so clearly that you feel the emotions of achievement and your mood changing. Visualising a positive experience will inadvertently have a positive effect on your biochemistry, lifting your spirits and your vibration instantly.

Step 6. Continue to visualise, focusing completely on what you can see and how it is making you feel. Allow this feeling to wash over you.

Step 7. Apply consistency. This needs to become a daily discipline to be effective. Your desire for this positive outcome will grow as your mind and body work towards bringing it to fruition.

The practice of both meditation and visualisations can be combined and take just 20 minutes a day, once the practice is a habit. The benefits are not only vast, but are scientifically proven. This simple discipline is easy to implement yet it can reap huge rewards in terms of mental and physical health, as well as increasing your belief in achieving the desired outcome. Explore the power of your mind by setting aside a little time every day to implement this discipline. Greater results are achieved over time. What answers lie within you? Invest a little time daily to find out.

ACTION POINTS

• Use the seven small steps to calmness to begin your daily meditation practice

• End each meditation with a vivid visualisation of a positive outcome that you would like to achieve

• Apply consistency to these daily disciplines, setting aside a little time to practise for the next 30 days

• Notice the gradual changes to your mind and body as a result of this new and rewarding habit

THE POWER OF THE SUBCONSCIOUS MIND

*'What the mind can conceive and
believe, it can achieve'*
NAPOLEON HILL

This chapter will help if you:

• Want to know how you built your internal and
external belief system

• Have underestimated the power of your
subconscious mind

• Want a tool kit to change thinking patterns and
habits

Most of us are aware that we have a conscious and subconscious
mind but few fully understand the difference, so we hugely
underestimate the power of the subconscious mind.

The conscious mind is where most people live day by day, but
it only equates to 10% of our total mind. This part of the mind is
your awareness of the present moment. It can only hold one
thought at a time; therefore it has no space to store memory. The
conscious mind has the ability to be critical of suggestion and it

can make comparisons between the possible actions that one might take.

The subconscious mind takes up 90% of our total mind, and many experts believe that we only use 3% of it. The subconscious mind stores all our learning and experiences. It also holds the key to our automated functions and reflexes, such as driving and walking. It is a huge memory bank with a virtually unlimited capacity, storing everything that has ever happened to us. By the time you turn 21, your mind has already stored more than 100 times the contents of the *Encyclopaedia Britannica*. Under hypnosis, it is not unusual for clients to recall, with perfect clarity, certain events that they had long forgotten about. These memories are buried deep in their subconscious, easily accessible through hypnotherapy.

Data is continually stored and retrieved by your subconscious, which is programming your belief system and instigating your responses, keeping you thinking and behaving in a manner according to your past experiences.

A simple example of this is driving. Remember when you were learning to drive? You had to think about every single part of the process. You would have had a conscious awareness of when to look in the mirror, use the indicator and change gear. Once driving is a daily habit, this skill set becomes automated and is then stored in your subconscious mind. If you are a regular driver, it is highly likely that you have frequently entered into 'highway hypnosis'. This is when you arrive at your destination with little recollection of the route you took, the songs that were on the car radio or any of the driving process. Highway hypnosis occurs because all of your driving skills are stored in your subconscious mind, where they have become automated and require hardly any conscious thinking.

The subconscious mind likes the stable equilibrium of homeostasis in both the mind and body. In the body, it has a role in stabilising body temperature, breathing patterns and heart rate via the autonomic nervous system. In the mind, it keeps your thinking patterns and behaviours consistent with past experiences in an effort to maintain homeostasis by keeping you comfortable.

Between the conscious and the subconscious mind is where the conscious critical faculty (CCF) resides. The CCF is a filter, which enables us to compare a situation with our belief system. The conscious mind will use the CCF to assess whether a situation can be dealt with by the subconscious or if it is an entirely new experience. The subconscious mind will cause you to feel emotionally and physically uncomfortable whenever you attempt to do anything new or different, or if you attempt to over-ride established patterns of behaviour. This is what is often referred to as 'stepping outside your comfort zone', something that your subconscious will pull you back towards each time you try something new or different. This part of the mind is the reason that we feel insecure, anxious and fearful on our first day of school, first day at a new job, doing something we have never attempted before or have an unsuccessful memory of, such as public speaking or dating.

Obviously as we go through life we are increasing the number of experiences stored in our subconscious. This data is our belief system and is made up of information that our subconscious has deemed necessary for survival – even our fears and phobias are initially conceived to 'protect' us. The content of our belief system falls into two categories; external and internal beliefs.

External beliefs are created when we accept and take on board things that other people have discovered. Languages, religions and cultural influences are all examples of external beliefs.

Internal beliefs are acquired as we grow, and are associated with the belief that we have in ourselves. This part of our belief system is largely built by the way that we are treated by others. Repetitive behaviour or language used towards us will serve to strengthen our inner belief system, whether it is self-esteem building or self-esteem destroying. Primarily, our internal beliefs are created by parents, siblings, teachers, bosses and figures in authority. Unfortunately, when we take on board beliefs that damage our self-esteem we may not appreciate that they have been passed on to us by people who are basing their actions and comments on their own belief system, which was created in exactly the same way. A cycle is therefore created, be it negative or positive. If a concept or belief is repeated to us from an early age it will form part of our belief system. A positive example of this is being consistently told that you are clever and have potential to succeed, which increases self-esteem, self-belief and acceptance. A negative example is being told that you will never get far in life and are a disappointment, which induces low self-esteem, insecurity and feelings of not being good enough.

Our internal belief system becomes a self-fulfilling prophecy, where we portray ourselves in alignment with our beliefs.

Furthermore, if others affirm the belief, one accepts and cements it. However if one is told the opposite, one's CCF will throw the suggestion out as being 'untrue'. An example is that if your parents divorce and you have an unfaithful partner yourself, the subconscious would have received the message that committed relationships rarely work. An internal belief is created that you risk being hurt if you allow yourself to get close to someone. Your CCF will then reject any comment or feeling that involves 'commitment'.

It is now easy to see how our personalities, habits, fears, morals and values are moulded and shaped through our life experiences. We often question the actions of ourselves and others, failing to understand the behaviour of others, and are critical of their conduct, particularly when we are on the receiving end. Try to recognise that all behaviour is a reflection of the inner belief system, and that unfavourable actions are an indication that the person is fighting an internal battle that even they may not fully understand.

The good news is that the CCF can be bypassed on certain occasions, which allows for short-term suspension or long-term changes of the internal belief system in the subconscious mind. An example of short-term suspension would be reading a fantasy novel or watching a superhero film. Our subconscious mind knows that it is unsafe to jump from a high-rise building, but while we watch *Superman* we are fully accepting of his flying abilities.

Bypassing the CCF quickly under hypnosis can make long-term changes to the subconscious mind. The National Hypnotherapy Society explains this as,

*'A completely natural state of consciousness in
which the conscious critical faculty is bypassed and
acceptable selective thinking is established.'*

In my hypnotherapy clinic, I have had excellent results with clients who are experiencing an inner conflict between their on-going behaviour and the behaviour that they would like to exhibit. Under hypnosis this inner conflict can be resolved.

One particular client named Jessica came to my clinic for help with alcohol intake. She realised that alcohol had become a coping mechanism she was using to escape from the stresses of her everyday life, which included marital issues and feelings of inadequacy. Jessica had been a barmaid, and had therefore spent much time with people who used alcohol to numb their problems. When Jessica's marriage experienced problems her subconscious told her that alcohol would provide evasion from these issues. Weekend drinking evolved into weekday drinking, and before long Jessica had lost her job due to her lack of attendance.

Jessica explained that she wanted desperately to change her behaviour because not only was she beginning to suffer health implications, but her family was concerned for her wellbeing and she knew in her heart that this behaviour was not resolving anything, in fact, it was making things far worse. This was a crucial factor in the success of Jessica's hypnotherapy, as you cannot manipulate the subconscious to do something it does not want to do. However, Jessica had expressed her desire to change, which meant that her inner conflict could be resolved under hypnotherapy. It took a single session of hypnotherapy, lasting 45 minutes to bring about the change Jessica was unable to make herself. This was achieved by suspending the CCF using progressive muscle relaxation techniques to allow me to access the subconscious mind without objection. Here I was able to resolve the inner conflict and insert positive suggestions and appropriate coping mechanisms for the future. Once I brought Jessica out of hypnosis, I spoke to her about the importance of reaffirming the work that we had done in the subconscious mind with daily affirmations. Together we decided that the best affirmations for her were:

'I am happy, healthy and enjoying my life', 'I am all I need to overcome any situation', and 'I am proud of myself and my achievements'.

I rarely contact clients for a progress update after hypnotherapy as I feel that it indicates doubt in the success of the treatment long-term. Instead, I simply invite my clients to 'keep in touch'.

I was delighted to hear from Jessica eight weeks after her treatment, when she phoned to tell me she had not had any alcohol for the entire duration, had coped without her usual crutch when quarrelling with her husband, had met friends in a pub and ordered soft drinks only, and had been on a family holiday without missing alcohol.

Never underestimate the power of the subconscious mind, because it has a largely untapped potential. Any limiting beliefs within our internal belief system have been built by us to keep us 'safe' and in our comfort zone. If this programming is no longer serving you, it is possible to change it, and as Jessica and many others have learnt, you can change your mind and change your *life*.

The placebo effect is a perfect example of just how powerful the subconscious mind is capable of being. Also called the placebo response this is a remarkable phenomenon, explained by Dr David Hamilton in his ground-breaking book, How Your Mind Can Heal Your Body. A placebo is a fake treatment or inactive substance which can improve a patient's condition simply because the person has the expectation that it will be helpful.

To illustrate the power of the subconscious mind further, consider pseudocyesis, also known as phantom pregnancies, which can occur in some woman due to psychological reasons. When a woman has a phantom pregnancy, her subconscious mind causes cessation of menstruation, breast enlargement, strange food cravings, progressive abdominal enlargement and even labour pains. Furthermore, some doctors, dentists and therapists have used hypnosis for medical purposes. Dr James Esdaile, a Scottish surgeon practising in the 1800s used hypnotism in operations before anaesthesia was available. He also planted suggestions in their subconscious minds to facilitate healing. In 161 operations performed by Dr Esdaile using hypnosis, the mortality rate was 5%, compared to the 50% average at that time.

Hypnotherapy can be a fast and often effortless way to re-programme your internal belief system and it is easier than you think to benefit from the power of your subconscious mind and give up limiting beliefs. There are also other ways to achieve this that may not be as quick as hypnotherapy, but can be just as effective when used as a daily discipline over time. Robert Collier, the American author of self-help and metaphysical books wrote,

'One comes to believe whatever one repeats to oneself sufficiently often, whether the statement be true or false.'

This is a perfect explanation of the subconscious mind working through recognised patterns and habits, which is why we can often go into autopilot with highly repetitive tasks. This is also the reason why daily affirmations, written well and repeated daily will bring about positive changes in your internal belief system and subsequently change your behaviour. Affirmations are a sure-fire way to silence self-doubt when integrated into your daily routine.

This quote from Martha Washington, wife of the US president, George Washington, serves as a stark reminder that we are the gatekeepers of our subconscious mind and have the power and tools to take control of our thoughts, feelings, internal belief system and overall the positivity of our mindset;

'I am still determined to be cheerful and happy, in whatever situation I may be; for I have also learned from experience that the greater part of our happiness or misery depends upon our dispositions, and not upon our circumstances.'
MARTHA WASHINGTON

Unleash the power inside your subconscious mind by surrendering the internal beliefs that no longer serve you and are holding you back. The subconscious mind has been trying to keep you in your comfort zone, as it thought you would be safe there, but as we all know, outside your comfort zone is where the 'magic' happens. Commit to re-programming your subconscious mind with the implementation of a few simple daily disciplines which are easy to do and can create big shifts in your life over time. Train your brain to create the 'sparkle effect' –

AFFIRMATIONS + GRATITUDE + POSITIVITY = SPARKLE EFFECT

ACTION POINTS

- Make a list of the limiting internal beliefs or inner conflicts that you have

- Write affirmations to assist you in reprogramming your internal beliefs and say them at least once a day

- Cultivate an attitude of gratitude with a daily gratitude list or journal

- Embrace the power of positivity and enjoy the sparkle effect

LET IT GO

'Be like a tree, let the dead leaves drop'
RUMI

This chapter will help if you:

- Often find yourself making comparisons with other people

- Feel overwhelmed by the things you think you need to change

- Are controlled by fear and consumed by negativity

We are all unique beings who experience life in completely different ways. The relationships and experiences that we have make us who we are and help to create our inner belief system, often without us even realising. It isn't until we decide to bring awareness to our thought process that we realise we are harbouring multiple imprints that do not serve us, yet we hold on to them because they are familiar.

Our beliefs either empower us, or limit us. While many of the beliefs we have acquired serve us well, some are simply habituated patterns continuing to produce the same unwanted outcomes. The human brain has an evolutionary tendency to remember and emphasise negative experiences.

Do you ever find yourself feeling fearful, resentful, angry, worried, guilty, frustrated or anxious? Do you compare yourself to other people? Do you have punishing expectations of yourself? All these emotions will be built upon an experience that has left the impression of an expected outcome. You are most likely to feel them when you fear that you are losing control of a situation.

Arguably, the deepest need we have is for a sense of control. When we feel out of control, we experience a powerful and uncomfortable **tension**. Considering that control is so significant to our emotions, why do we become so concerned with things that are beyond our control?

Patricia Carrington PhD, author of *The Power of Letting Go*, writes,

> *'Letting go of our insistence on controlling what is beyond our reach is a key to peace of mind.'*

In this chapter, you will learn how to go from fear to freedom by releasing what does not serve you, allowing you to find your own inner reality and peace.

Learning to let go of thoughts, feelings, or relationships that are no longer conducive to your wellbeing is fundamental for your overall health. This practice is a detox for the mind, which is possibly the most toxic part of our body, and one that is often overlooked on traditional detox plans.

A recurring conversation that I have with clients regarding both the mind and body is how to handle being overwhelmed. Many have told me that they live in fear of not being able to make all the changes they feel they need to in order to reach their goal. This is living in fear of not being good enough, or not being accepted or validated by others. These are not emotions or feelings that serve and they need to be released. In speaking to clients about where these feelings stem from and how they are aggravated, a common theme emerged. It seems that many of us compare ourselves with others, a habit made far easier now that we have a direct window into other people's lives through social media. Clients have told me that after a short glance through Facebook and Instagram they can feel anxious, upset and inadequate for the remainder of the day. It would serve us all well to remember that the majority of social media posts are personal branding and self-advertisement, whether they are contrived or not. While some people do share the downsides to life on these platforms, most only show 'the best bits', much like a film trailer. Social media, whether negative or positive, is not a true representation of one's life. Feeling anxious and inadequate because of what you have seen on social media is the equivalent of comparing your body to that of a mannequin, which has been shaped and moulded to fit an image or perception.

Negative emotions (anger, sadness, frustration, fear, anxiety, jealousy, low self-esteem) that we hold inside can sometimes be an even greater cause of stress, and eventually chronic disease.

Dr Candace Pert, the innovative American neuroscientist who

founded mind-body medicine, and wrote *The Molecules of Emotion*, said,

> '*Your mind is in every cell of your body. A feeling sparked in your mind will translate as a peptide being released somewhere. Peptides regulate every aspect of your body, from whether your going to digest your food properly to whether you are going to destroy a tumour cell.*'

Dr Pert is responsible for decades of research, 250 scientific research papers and two best-selling books. Consider that your thoughts and emotions are impacting your health, and commit to taking action to ensure that the impact is a positive one.

The first step towards letting go of the things that no longer serve you is to identify what is holding you back, keeping you in a negative place and ultimately affecting your health. This exercise will take time, patience and a lot of self-exploring, but it is not something that has to be completed in one sitting. Take as long as you need, as the peace and self-love it can bring is truly worthy of the work.

When I decided to start this practice, I bought a notebook and took half an hour each day to detox my mind of any negativity I felt I was harbouring. Of course, you do not have to do it this way, if you are more visual, you may prefer just to close your eyes and use visualisations. It is also important to point out that we are not attempting to create a sterile mindset free from all negativity, as that is impossible to maintain. This is about bringing balance to your mind's thoughts so that they are not over-powered by affliction.

In my daily half an hour, I brought awareness to some of the reoccurring thoughts that brought about a negative emotion whenever they crossed my mind. The most obvious and overpowering reflection that often replayed in my mind was the loss of my mum. I realised that this was making me feel guilty because I couldn't help her. I was ashamed of the times I wished she was no longer suffering, resentful of people around me who still had their mother and fearful that it may happen to me. But how could I just let go of that much hurt and heal that deep a wound?

I started by writing down a list of the negative emotions that this thought brought me, and realised that none of these were serving me in any way. You may argue that these were all part of the grieving process, but I believe they were simply keeping me stuck in grief.

I then asked myself if I could change this situation or whether it was beyond my control. Obviously, in this instance, there was nothing I could do to reverse my loss, however, there was lots that I could do to cope with the constant wave of negative thoughts.

I looked at all the negative thoughts written in my notebook that were linked to the loss of my mum and wrote an opposing statement for each one.

Next to 'guilty: because I couldn't help her', I wrote; 'I didn't have the knowledge that I have now to improve her quality or quantity of life. This is frustrating, but I am now able to use my knowledge to help others. I did everything I possibly could to help my mum at the time and I have no reason to feel any guilt.'

I continued this process for each negative emotion, each time providing a reason to let go of the pattern of thinking that was only causing me to feel a mixture of toxic emotions.

> 'Your worst enemy can not harm you as much as
> your own unguarded thoughts'
> BUDDHA

Reading my statement back I realised how unkind I had been to myself. Would I tell a grieving friend that they should have done more? Absolutely not! So why wasn't I treating myself with the same level of respect. I believe we are all guilty of being our own worst enemies, listening to negative self-talk and developing self-limiting beliefs. This is unkind, unnecessary and will lead to poor physical and mental health. We all need to become our own best friends, giving ourselves the same level of kindness that we show others. This is not something that can happen overnight, as we have a lifetime of bad behaviour to change. Knowing how destructive this conduct can be and learning to recognise and reframe it is an infinite, on-going effort, but it serves to encourage self-love and optimise wellbeing.

By noting down the negative emotions I was feeling, and bringing an awareness to their origins, I had set my intent to journey from fear to freedom. Each day I found a small amount of time to get inside my own mind and decipher my feelings, guard my thoughts and continually detox my mind. As this process became a daily discipline I begun to feel lighter, happier and more energised.

Although this was initially a daily habit, I now only use the process as a form of mind maintenance. If I feel the balance of my thoughts tip towards negativity or my feelings become overwhelmingly heavy, I take time to investigate, reason and release all that does not serve me.

The last entry I made into my notebook reads: 'my insecurities are making me feel anxious'. After careful consideration, thinking back to the last few occasions that I felt insecure, I wrote the following statement; 'I am a very sensitive people-pleaser who seeks validation and acceptance from others. There is no need to focus on what other people think of me. I need no validation or acceptance as I am already enough. It is impossible to please everyone and not everyone will like me, that is fine. I will make peace with who I am and what I have to offer and let go of my need for validation and outside approval.'

Since writing this statement, I have caught myself feeling fear and anxiety after a 'what if they don't like me' moment. I simply remember my statement, whisper I am enough and let go of this unproductive thought. The fact is if someone doesn't like me, there is little I can do about it, since it is out of my control. The irony is, by accepting this I feel more in control than ever before.

As the character Elsa in the Disney film *Frozen*, said,

*'The fear that once controlled me, can't get to me at
all. No right, no wrong, no rules for me. I'm free.'*

From working with clients and by working on my own mind detox
I have realised that many of us carry guilt or shame for what we
consider to be our failings. Actually, when you look a little closer
at these so-called failings, it is just the way we have framed them,
so reframing helps us to let go.

I also come across many people who, like me, are dwelling on
what they should have done or could have done. The 'should,
would, could and what if' mindset is highly toxic because it is
referencing a past event that cannot be changed or rectified.
However, we can reframe our thinking by accepting 'what's done
is done' and letting go of the things that we cannot alter to bring
focus, clarity and direction to the things that we can change.

Five hundred years ago, the French philosopher, Michel de
Montaigne said,

*'My life has been filled with terrible misfortune;
most of which never happened.'*

A 1996 study carried out by Adrian Wells of the University of
Manchester and Gerald Matthews of the University of Cincinnati,
concluded that 85% of what we worry about never materialises.
This suggests that we are putting the health of our mind and body
at risk for no good reason.

Learning to access, analyse and release negative thoughts and emotions may seem arduous and time-consuming, but so is going to the gym. We appear to invest time and money in training our body but do not make the same effort with our mind, which can be just as dangerous if left unchecked. If you would like to learn more on emotional and mental resilience, I recommend reading *The Power of Neuroplasticity* by Shad Helmstetter PhD.

Take action to restore your health and happiness by dedicating a little time to declutter your mind, letting go of all that does not serve you to allow and accept all that does.

ACTION POINTS

- Take time each day to acknowledge your negative thoughts and feelings

- Dissolve negativity by realising how much of your worries are beyond your control

- Let go of what you cannot change to focus on what you can

- Remember that social media is a film trailer, so be kind to yourself by remaining comparison-free

YOUR VIBE, YOUR TRIBE

*'If you want to find the secrets of the universe, think
in terms of energy, frequency and vibrations'*
NIKOLA TESLA

This chapter will help if you:

• Feel like you don't 'fit in'

• Are surrounded by people who bring you down

• Want to know how to raise your vibration to
  attract your tribe

The worst kind of loneliness is feeling alone in a crowd. I know
this because I have felt it many times.

I used to have a group of 'friends' that I had known for a
considerable amount of time. Whenever I was around them I felt
anxious, inferior and inadequate, I never truly understood what
made me feel this way and at the time I blamed myself and other
external factors. I would wonder if I felt isolated because I wasn't
in the same income bracket, with the same number of designer
shoes or handbags, and in some way was not validated. Anytime
that I was due to go out with them I would work myself into a

frenzy over what to wear and what to talk about, and I was a bundle of nervous energy.

When I lost my mother these same people did not come to her funeral, call me or even send a message of condolence, which is when I had the realisation that these people were not my *tribe*.

It took the loss of my mum to realise that your value doesn't decrease based on someone's inability to see your worth, and that you never really lose friends, you simply find out who your true ones are. Those who are attracted to you because of what you have or look like will not be by your side forever. Neither will the ones who make you feel inferior for what you don't have, or anxious because you fail to fit into their mould of perfection. It's the people who can see how beautiful your heart is who will never leave your life, and regardless of your success or failures they will walk beside you in a non-judgemental and completely unconditional way.

I feel incredibly grateful and blessed to have replaced the dogmatic and materialistic group I knew before with kind, heart-centred people who love me fiercely. The depth of their love has taken me on a journey of fundamental truths of spirituality and consciousness. They are my tribe.

If I had not lost my mum when I did, maybe I would still have the same kind of people in my life. As I said before, the worst possible experiences can often put you on the path to the best. Even without this devastating loss, I'm sure that I would have eventually tired of those people and the way that I felt when I was with them. In the immediate aftermath of my parents' deaths, I only really had one friend who supported me in my darkest hours, to whom I will always be grateful. I noticed that I was attracting new people into my life who had also been through loss and grief, and I even received a letter from a school mum I had never spoken to, telling me about the loss of her own mother ten years previously. She was offering her support and I was touched that she took the time to reach out when she hardly knew me, especially when so many long-standing friends had failed to do so. It made me realise that I needed to change my vibration to attract the positive and uplifting tribe that I was missing.

In accordance with the universal Law of Attraction, you attract into your life the people, circumstances and things that correspond with your dominant, habitual thoughts. The thoughts and feelings that you vibrate are what the Universe echoes back to you, known as 'sympathetic vibrations'. The universal law of vibration also has a role in what you are attracting. This law states that everything in the Universe moves, travels and vibrates in circular patterns, including our thoughts, feelings and words. If you are in any doubt about these universal laws, have you ever been having a seriously bad day but tried hard to hide it? Then someone says, 'Smile! It might never happen!' They have picked up on your negative vibrations, and this is a skill we all have. Dr Bernard Beitman, former chairman of the department of psychiatry at the US University of Missouri-Columbia and graduate of Yale Medical School looks at studies of the brain and energy emitted by living beings to hypothesise about the physical nature of vibes. He says,

'Our bodies have receptors to pick up on this energy'

In addition, the behaviour analyst Jessica Stephans says,

> *'Animals secrete hormones that others instinctively respond to, so why wouldn't it be the same for humans?'*

Still doubting the power of vibrational energy? Please take the time to watch Dr Masaru Emoto's rice experiment on YouTube. Dr Emoto, a Japanese author and researcher, placed three cups of rice in water. For the next month he said, 'thank you' to one cup, 'you are an idiot' to the second and he completely ignored the third. The result was that after 30 days the rice that had been thanked began to ferment, giving off a pleasant aroma. The rice that had been insulted turned black, and the rice that had been ignored began to rot. It's an interesting experiment that is easy to do at home, especially to teach children that words and negative energy are harmful to everything in its field.

If you are thinking that 'vibes' is a hippy term that belongs in the Woodstock era, I'm sure you have experienced picking up on a good or bad energy around a particular person or place. This is their vibration and you will know instantly if it matches yours. If it doesn't and you stay around, be prepared to have your vibration changed to fall into alignment with your surroundings. When you feel as if the people you're with only lift you higher, you are likely to have found your *tribe*.

If you are in the position that I once was and feel that you are not attracting the right kind of people, you need to raise your

YOUR VIBE, YOUR TRIBE

vibration. In doing so you will begin to attract a group whose consciousness matches yours.

Rebecca Campbell, fellow lightworker and author of *Light is the New Black* and *Rise Sister Rise* says,

> *'It doesn't take a big action to increase your vibration'*

I couldn't agree more. Your vibration can be raised rapidly and it can remain high with the use of consistent healthy habits and daily disciplines. Use the following top tips to become the energy that you want to attract.

TOP TEN TIPS TO RAISE YOUR VIBRATION

1. Show Gratitude and Appreciation

Having an Attitude of Gratitude can ignite the power of positivity and instantly raise your vibration from one of lack, wanting and need to abundance, grateful and blessed.

2. Make Healthy Food Choices

Listen to your body and pay attention to how foods make you feel. Food is either feeding illness or wellness, and a diseased body will struggle to raise vibrations. Choose foods that raise your energy levels and leave you feeling nourished (see Clean Eating and Proper Preparation chapters).

3. Decrease Your Toxic Load

The levels of toxicity in your body will have a direct impact on your energy, concentration, mood and overall health. A happy, energised person will radiate positive vibrations. Also consider detoxing from social media or certain people that lower your vibration (refer to the Decrease Your Toxic Load chapter for further guidance).

4. Do Meditation and Visualisations

We live in a busy world, full of noise and pressure, which can lower your vibration through stress and anxiety. Taking a little time out daily to meditate, or simply just visualising a peaceful place, your goals or loved ones can release the tension of daily life and instantly raise your vibration. Refer to the Meditation and Visualisation chapter for further guidance.

5. Repeat Affirmations

As explained by Dr David Hamilton PhD in his book, *How Your Mind Can Heal Your Body*, when we repeat a statement we create neural connections in our brain. Repeating daily positive affirmations will change neural pathways, brain activity and thought patterns to lead you towards your goals. Affirmations create positive energy and positive energy raises vibrations.

6. Carry Out Random Acts of Kindness

Being kind will instantly lift your vibration and leave you feeling great. As Princess Diana said, *'Carry out a random act of kindness, with no expectation of reward, safe in the knowledge that one day someone might do the same for you.'* Abundance not only creates a higher vibration, but it will be returned to you via the universal law of compensation that states the effects of our deeds are returned to us.

7. Practice Forgiveness

Harbouring negative thoughts or feelings about someone who has upset you in the past is toxic to your mind and body. Understand that everybody has imperfections and carrying anger, hurt or shame will only keep you in a low vibration. If you feel that reconciliation isn't possible, simply let go of the resentment and any desire for revenge. Psychologists have found that those who can make this mental shift are rewarded with a longer and happier life.

8. Get Moving

Exercise releases chemicals in the brain known as endorphins, which trigger positive, uplifting feelings. Find the exercise you enjoy the most, even if it is something as simple as dancing to your favourite song. Get your blood pumping, endorphins flowing and vibrations raised (refer to the HIIT chapter for tips on exercising).

9. Use a Himalayan Salt Lamp

Salt lamps give out negative ion particles, which purify the air and neutralise the damaging positive ions produced through electromagnetic fields, fluorescent lights and air pollution. Negative ions also elevate our mood by increasing serotonin levels, help to stabilise blood pressure, increase the body's alkalinity, strengthen bones, heighten immunity and accelerate physical recovery. Negative ions are abundant in nature, so getting out into the fresh air is also hugely beneficial but when inside, using a Himalayan salt lamp will raise the positive vibrations in your home, safeguarding your health and mood.

10. Have Faith

85% of the things that we worry about never actually happen. So many of our concerns are out of our control, which is why worrying makes no difference to the overall outcome. Worry will never take away tomorrow's troubles; instead it will take today's peace. Don't allow worry to lower your vibration, instead have utter faith and trust in the Universe. Life coach and author Gabrielle Bernstein documents how to transform fear into faith in her best-selling book *The Universe Has Your Back*, and says, 'the key to serenity is trusting that the universe has your back.' Worrying never changed an outcome but it will change your vibration. Have faith that there is a divine plan for you already mapped out, and simply enjoy the journey. Releasing the burden of worry will raise your vibration (the chapter Let It Go may help with this).

Looking back at my experience of not fitting in and feeling as if I wasn't accepted, it is now clear why. I was trying to be someone else in order to be accepted by a group of people that I didn't have much in common with. It's little wonder that I didn't fit in and felt so lonely in their presence. Be true to yourself and 100% authentic or you will attract a tribe that does not resonate with you, your values or your level of consciousness. If the people you are spending time with are making you feel excluded or withdrawn, it is time to honour your emotions, raise your vibrations and attract your true tribe, a group of like-minded beings who you have a natural connection with rather than a forced one.

Social influence makes us all more similar to the people we spend time with. We can't *help* but conform to some degree, or for the ideals of our peers to blend with our own. This is one of the reasons it is so important to find your tribe, without them you will dilute your own opinions to win acceptance, which will become draining and ultimately cause resentment.

You will know instantly that you have found your tribe because you can be *you* again. The people around you will take you as you are, they will likely share in your interests but if they don't, they will definitely share the same values and moral compass. They will be the first to congratulate you when you succeed, but equally pick you up and dust you down without judgement or ridicule when you don't. These people will not simply tolerate you; they will celebrate you and be as thankful to know you, as you are glad to know them. When you are surrounded by those that provide you with uplifting energy instead of draining it (radiators instead of drains), your vibration will be higher with very little effort.

Stick with the people who pull the magic out of you, and who allow you to shine bright like the star that you are. You will not only attract other stars, but you will light the way for those who are in darkness.

ACTION POINTS

- Assess whether you are surrounded by people who lift you higher. Are they radiators or drains?

- Use the Top Ten Tips to raise your vibration and become the energy that you want to attract

- Have love and gratitude for your newfound self-acceptance and your tribe

- Keep your vibrations high to attract other tribe members and to light the way for those in darkness

YOU ARE ENOUGH

*'Realise how amazing you are. All
you have to do is be yourself'*
ANITA MOORJANI

This chapter will help if you:

- Are a people-pleaser, constantly seeking
  validation from others

- Look outside yourself for answers and solutions

- Move the goal posts and strive for perfection

We live in a world where it seems as if we are constantly being measured and judged in some way. In our personal lives, we post pictures on social media and await 'likes' and comments. In our working lives, we are appraised by our employers to determine whether we have worked hard enough and are worthy of reward. Whether it is seeking praise as a parent or acceptance from friends, I'm sure there will be some part of you that craves validation from others. If I am honest, this is something that I continually need to work on in my own personal journey of self-acceptance and self-love.

Self-love is the foundation of inner happiness, and you have to love yourself to be able to love others because you cannot give what you do not have. In the development of complete self-love and self-belief, you will no longer look to other people to fill a void, as you realise that approval and validation is unnecessary from anyone other than yourself.

This level of self-acceptance and love is when you know that you are enough, even with perfect imperfections, flaws and weaknesses – you are still enough. Reaching this realisation does not mean that you finally measured up and gained approval from the judges, nor does it mean that you will never need to ask for help or guidance again. Knowing and believing that you are enough is accepting that you are on a journey and you have everything you need for this journey within. You don't have to *prove* yourself, you just need to *be* yourself. Unapologetically *you*.

A place of self-love and acceptance free from judgement and criticism sounds like a blissful space to be in. However, to get there, we first must silence our inner critic.

We all live with a 'Negative Nancy' or 'Nigel'. You know that inner voice that is constantly critical, telling us that we aren't good enough. It is listening to this internal critic that assists in the development of limiting beliefs and self-sabotaging behaviour. It is so easy to get stuck in our own heads as our inner critic tears apart our self-esteem because we didn't make the grade in some way. We are our own worst enemies, judging and criticising ourselves in a relentless way that we would never do to others, readily dismissing all the unique and wonderful attributes that we have.

Learning to silence that inner critic as you journey to self-love and freedom from validation is an on-going process in an effort to keep that 'Negative Nancy' in check. Even with self-development and awareness it is far too easy to allow the negative talk to return. It only takes a derogatory comment directed at you or a quick scroll through social media to see all of those perfect 'selfies', to make us feel inferior and not 'good enough'. Then the voice of Nancy: 'Maybe you should get your nose done' or "You shouldn't have skipped that last gym session' or 'You will never do as well in your career as them' or 'Why aren't your kids winning awards at school?'. It goes on and on, and most of the time we aren't even fully aware of what we are doing and the damage it is causing.

As I mentioned, social media is like a film trailer, and mostly shows only the best parts of people's lives. It is self-advertisement and self-validation in the highest form. I'm not against it, as I use it for both business and pleasure, but I encourage you to be a mindful user, taking its content with a pinch of salt. As for 'selfies', here's what I initially thought: 'Wow, how confident must one be to continually post selfies?' Here's what I later realised, 'Wow, how much validation does one crave to post selfies continuously?' #livingforlikes

You see, everyone has insecurities, even selfie addicts. In fact, I would hazard a guess that they may be experiencing a deep-rooted insecurity and are using selfies to bolster their self-esteem.

Often, it is the people that appear to be the most confident who are fighting an internal battle. Those who are quick to criticise and judge others often do so because they are trying to divert attention from the flaws they feel they have. You cannot show love and kindness to others if you do not first show it to yourself. In a world where we are being constantly judged, seeking acceptance and striving for perfection, we need to accept more and judge less. Perfection doesn't exist, so searching and striving for it is a fast route to unfulfillment and unhappiness. Accepting that you are enough, right now, as you are, without validation, without recognition and without acceptance from anyone other than yourself is a better alternative.

The journey of self-love starts with acknowledging your negative self-talk and learning to silence the inner critic by replacing it with an inner support system – your own inner cheerleader. In the Your Vibe, Your Tribe chapter I explain the immense value in finding a close inner circle of friends who unconditionally love and accept you. However, the process of attracting your tribe starts from within. It is enriching to have true friends who guide you from darkness back to light, but it is empowering to be able to do this yourself too.

The American self-help author Louise Hay says,

> *'You have been criticizing yourself for years,*
> *and it hasn't worked. Try approving of*
> *yourself and see what happens.'*

The answers are within. When we are feeling down we often look for external validation to lift our spirits, such as seeking compliments or looking for support from friends and relatives. It is important to be able to self-sooth to depend less on validation from others and begin that journey to self-love. Below are my eight practices to become your own support system:

1. Say it yourself!

Before seeking external support ask yourself what you are hoping to hear, and say it to yourself. It doesn't lose meaning if it comes from you, in fact it means more, as it is a true indication that you value your internal opinion more than an external one.

2. Judge less and accept more

Don't be so hard on yourself. Accept that you are exactly where you are supposed to be in life right now. Let go of all of the comparisons you make – this is your life and your journey. There is only one you and you are enough. Once you learn not to judge and to accept yourself, you will notice you treat others with the same level of respect.

3. Sit with it

Have you ever asked yourself 'Why am I feeling like this? Why can't I just be happy?' It's okay, we all do it sometimes, but this is judgement of our feelings. We can't be bouncing off the walls every day of the year, it's alright not to be okay, and in fact it's perfectly normal. Acknowledge your feelings and just sit with them for a while. Send yourself love and reassurance that this is not the final destination, just part of a journey. It will pass.

4. Address your needs

I have been prone to the occasional adult tantrum, which can leave me feeling guilty and ashamed about my behaviour. At these times we need to address our needs, just as we would with a child. Any moment of emotional instability will be triggered by a need not being met. It could be as simple as tiredness or hunger, as with children. It may be that you need to take a break, go for a walk, meditate to clear your mind, sleep or drink water. Addressing your needs is reinforcing self-love and validating yourself through your actions, as opposed to seeking validation from others.

5. Be proud of yourself

In the chapter An Attitude Of Gratitude, I detail the many benefits of keeping a daily gratitude journal to cultivate positivity. This is also a great place to harvest self-love by including a 'Proud of Me' list. Each day when writing your gratitude list, also write three things that you are proud of yourself for achieving in the last twenty-four hours. The more you practise self-praise and appreciation the less you will need to seek validation from external sources.

6. Affirm your worth

If you are lacking in self-confidence and self-esteem, include a confidence-boosting affirmation in your daily affirmations. It can be something as simple as 'I love and approve of myself. I am enough' Refer to the chapter on Daily Affirmations for a detailed account of how to write affirmations that resonate with you personally.

7. Love your inner child

Inside each of us is the child we once were. A child who meant no harm, tried their best, and simply wanted to please and be loved. There may have been occasions throughout childhood when that child did not receive the love, tenderness or support that they craved, which would have left a wound. This is the wound that can be linked to feelings of not being good enough. We carry these false beliefs with us and learn to reject ourselves. If you have experienced a traumatic childhood, I would recommend working with a therapist to heal your inner child and the hurts of the past. However, a simple exercise that we can all do is using visualisation, go back to your inner child and give them a hug. Tell them they are loved and that they have always been good enough. I have practiced this at times and it has led me to tears, so be prepared for this simple yet powerful technique.

8. Let go of validation goals

Clients often tell me that they know they will feel better when they get to their goal weight or get offered that promotion. They somehow believe that reaching this destination will define their worth. I have also had clients who have arrived in my office seeking hypnotherapy because they have reached their goal and still feel unworthy. Goal setting can be a positive thing, however, it should never have any emotion riding on it, especially your self-worth. If you do not believe you are enough before you achieve it, you still won't when you do achieve it.

Using these eight practices to become your own support system will allow you to replace the ever-lasting pursuit of perfection with contentment. Just imagine for one moment being free from feelings of comparison, inferiority, jealousy and judgement because you finally accepted that you are already enough. I would also like you to think of all the things these feelings have held you back from attempting. Fear of the opinions and criticism of others hold us back from reaching our true purpose. The inspiring author and public speaker Brene Brown once asked during a public speaking event, 'What would you try if you knew people would never say things about you?' When you give this question any thought at all, you will realise just how much you have valued the opinions of others.

It is safe to say that if you spend your life attempting to please others, you will spend it being someone you are not and will never fulfil your true purpose. I believe that we all have a purpose to fulfil, we are all a gift to this world. Some will not see your true worth and that is absolutely fine, so don't waste your precious time trying to convince them of it. Some will see your true worth but will not like it and may attempt to dim your shine, so don't focus on them. Many will not be meant for your path, as they are not supposed to be part of your journey, so convincing them to walk alongside you will only inflict unnecessary wounds. Rebecca Campbell writes in *Light is The New Black:*

'You are not for everyone and that's OK. Don't waste your precious time and gifts trying to convince them of your value, they won't ever want what you're selling.'

While some will attempt to dim your light, many others will see you for the shining star that you are, and will love you fiercely and unconditionally. These are the people who will hear you without needing convincing and the ones who are privileged to journey with you, building your self-belief instead of knocking it down.

Dr. Steve Maraboli is a life-changing speaker, bestselling author, and Behavioural Science academic. His empowering and insightful words have been shared and published throughout the world. This quote exemplifies all I have written in this chapter,

'You are a beautiful creation... perfectly imperfect...
a work in progress... you have everything you need
to fulfil your purpose... don't dilute yourself for any
person or any reason... you are enough...
be unapologetically you.'

Don't waste your time on waiting for validation and acceptance, gift the world with *you*. There is only one you, you are set apart from everyone else, unique and individual. You have been given everything you need to achieve what you desire and fulfil your purpose. Be true to who you are, believe in yourself, believe in your value and above all else believe that you are enough.

ACTION POINTS

- Listen out for your negative self-talk and take action to silence it

- Become your own biggest supporter, using some or all of the eight practices in this chapter

- Resist the urge to people-please; you do not need validation

- Believe with all your heart that you are already enough

BODY

FIGHT THE FIRE OF INFLAMMATION

'Your body's ability to heal is far, far greater than
you've ever been permitted to believe.'
MO ROSATI

This chapter will help if you:

- Suffer from an inflammatory condition such as
  arthritis or other autoimmune conditions

- Suffer with chronic pain and rely on medication to
  bring relief

- Want to know how your diet and lifestyle is
  impacting your health and more importantly how
  to change

Many people have a perception that inflammation within the
body is a negative reaction that needs to be overcome. With anti-
inflammatory medications and anti-inflammatory diets, we could
easily be coerced into thinking that inflammation is always
harmful. In actual fact it is a vital part of immunity, the body's
attempt to heal itself from injury; defend itself against foreign
invaders, such as viruses and bacteria; and repair damaged tissue.

If you were to sprain your ankle you would feel pain and see swelling and possibly redness. This is visible and external and is referred to as acute inflammation. It is merely the body transporting protective white blood cells to the area to commence the healing process. However, inflammation becomes an issue when it is invisible and internal. In this chapter we take a closer look at chronic internal inflammation, why it occurs, how to detect it and what diet and lifestyle measures we can take to reduce or eradicate it before it progresses into disease.

Chronic inflammation is long-term and as the title of this chapter suggests, it is like a fire raging inside your body. This type of inflammation occurs when the immune system becomes hyperactive in response to irritants such as smoking, stress, diet and medication. When the body is not healing because the stresses continue, the immune system will persevere in issuing an inflammatory response and eventually damage healthy tissue.

Chronic inflammation actually serves an important purpose within our bodies. It comes as a messenger for us to take stock and make changes to our diet and lifestyle. However, it is crucially important that we learn how to recognise these messages as they are a precursor to many chronic diseases.

There is a test that can be carried out to measure inflammation within the body called C-reactive protein (CRP). This is a blood test that I have performed on clients to assess their inflammation levels. High levels of CRP must be addressed in order to safeguard a client's health. Elevated CRP and cholesterol increase your risk of heart disease threefold. An eight-year study carried out on more than 28,000 women was published in the *New England Journal of Medicine* and found that more than 50% of the women who eventually developed heart disease had healthy levels of LDL bad cholesterol but high CRP levels. This demonstrates how CRP levels can be an indication of future health when other levels used to measure disease are regarded as safe.

However, it is not possible for everyone to test CRP levels in the body continually to protect their health. This is why it is vital to be able to recognise the signs of inflammation without a test in order to respond to the messages that your body is communicating.

An obvious sign of inflammation is persistent aches and pains in muscles and joints. Conditions such as fibromyalgia and arthritis are painful chronic inflammatory conditions, which cause on-going discomfort. Clients who have these conditions usually tell me they are learning to live with the pain, but why should they have to? Why should pain be a daily occurrence in someone's life? These particular conditions also fall into the autoimmune category. Excessive inflammation is a feature of all autoimmune diseases and is largely responsible for the symptoms common to many autoimmune conditions – pain, fatigue and poor quality sleep. If you have been diagnosed with an autoimmune disease you will most certainly be experiencing inflammation and I would encourage you to read this chapter, along with the chapter called Heal Your Gut to empower yourself with healing tools.

Allergies are another sign of inflammation, producing the most obvious symptoms of inflammation – swelling, redness, itching and pain. An allergic reaction is an over-reaction of the immune system, the body's natural defence system. The immune system responds to an allergen as though it's under attack, releasing antibodies and triggering inflammation, even though the stimulus of the attack (the allergen) is normally harmless.

Itchy skin and redness are also classic signs of inflammation, which can accompany autoimmune conditions or be caused by allergies or an unhealthy liver. An inflamed liver will produce much greater quantities of CRP and can become inflamed for a multitude of reasons.

Infections are a common cause of inflammation, particularly chronic infections that lie dormant. Some viruses and bacteria can remain in the body for years, including hepatitis C, Epstein Barr virus, herpes viruses and parasitic gut infections.

Excess body fat contributes to inflammation. As we gain weight our fat cells become enlarged as they fill with more fat. These cells may leak as they are stretched, so immune cells called 'macrophages' appear to clean the leakage. As the macrophages clean, they release inflammatory chemicals in the fatty tissues and it is this inflammatory response that may be behind many of the negative effects that being overweight has on a person's health.

It would be impossible to create an exhaustive list of inflammatory triggers because sources of inflammation are now so abundant in our environment, however your diet will be either feeding illness or wellness. The food and drink you are using to fuel your body may also be fuelling the inflammatory fire that is raging internally. Since acid is a precursor to inflammation, and inflammation is a precursor to disease, anti-inflammatory diets are also alkalising, in an attempt to reduce acid and improve inflammation before it goes on to become a disease.

Research entitled 'Diet-induced Acidosis', carried out in 2011, and published in *Clinical Nutrition* Volume 30, stated that a modern diet is devoid of alkalinity and the compounding effect of chronic acidosis leads to a host of problems in the body, including an increased risk of obesity, cardiovascular disease, diabetes, hypertension and chronic kidney failure.

To gain an understanding of the acidity level of your food choices, please study the pH chart below.

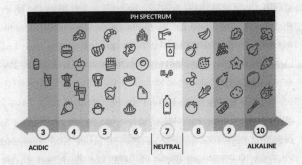

3. Carbonated Water, Club soda, Energy Drinks

4. Popcorn, Cream Cheese, Buttermilk, Prunes, Pastries, Pasta, Cheese, Pork, Beer, Wine, Black Tea, Pickles, Chocolate, Roasted Nuts, Vinegar, Sweet and Low, Equal, Nutra Sweet.

5. Most Purified Water, Distilled Water, Coffee, . Sweetened Fruit Juice, Pistachios, Beef, White Bread, Peanuts, Nuts, Wheat.

6. Fruit Juices, Most Grains, Eggs, Fish, Tea, Cooked Beans, Cooked Spinach, Soy Milk, Coconut, Lima Beans, Plums, Brown Rice, Barley, Cocoa, Oats, Liver, Oyster, Salmon.

7. Neutral pH - Most Tap Water, Most Spring Water, Sea Water, River Water.

8. Apples, Almonds, Tomatoes, Grapefruit, Corn, Mushrooms, Turnip, Olive, Soybeans, Peaches, Bell Pepper, Radish, Pineapple, Cherries, Wild Rice, Apricot, Strawberries, Bananas.

9. Avocados, Green Tea, Lettuce, Celery, Peas, Sweet Potatoes, Egg Plant, Green Beans, Beets, Blueberries, Pears, Grapes, Kiwi, Melons, Tangerines, Figs, Dates, Mangoes, Papayas.

10. Spinach, Broccoli, Artichoke, Brussel Sprouts, Cabbage, Cauliflower, Carrots, Cucumbers, Lemons, Limes, Seaweed, Asparagus, Kale, Radish, Collard Greens, Onion.

The most inflammatory foods are sugar, gluten, wheat, cow's milk, artificial additives and any food you have an allergy or intolerance to. A healthy, anti-inflammatory diet is based on vegetables, salads, protein (such as eggs, poultry, fish, meat, pulses), healthy fats, fruit, nuts and seeds. Try to avoid eating packaged foods. My easy-to-apply mantra for making food choices is, 'If it hasn't walked, swum, grew or flew, don't eat it!'

All food has a pH value, and the pH scale runs from 0 (pure acid) to 14 (most alkaline), with 7 being neutral. The human body functions optimally at a pH of around 7.4, which is just on the alkaline side of neutral. It is not difficult to see from the chart that a typical Western diet is composed predominantly of acid-forming foods. Stimulants such as tobacco, coffee, tea, and alcohol, as well as stress and inadequate physical activity are also extremely acidifying.

A body which is acidic will destroy its own cells, have a compromised immune system, accelerated ageing, difficulty in regulating metabolism and weight, be prone to disease and allergies, be nutrient-depleted, will not flush out toxins effectively, will not regulate cholesterol and will not maintain good oxygen levels.

Simply by reducing or eliminating acidic foods and replacing them with those that have an alkalizing effect, you will be reducing internal inflammation and decrease your chances of illness and disease.

The 'Get More' and 'Get Less' lists simplify the anti-inflammatory protocol:

Get More:

- Fresh foods
- Vegetables
- Fruits
- Nuts, seeds and pulses
- Salads
- Foods that are as close to nature (unrefined) as possible
- Filtered/purified water
- Exercise
- Fresh air
- Relaxation

Get Less:

- Sugar
- Fast foods and takeaway meals
- Junk foods and refined foods
- Excessive animal protein and dairy foods
- White foods (white bread, white pasta, etc)
- Caffeine
- Soft drinks and alcohol
- Stress and negative emotions

As a holistic health coach I have come up against opponents of an anti-inflammatory diet who state that reducing acid-forming foods in order to decrease inflammation is nothing more than pseudo-science. In response to this, I would like to share two things. Firstly, here is a quote by Dr Keiichi Morishita taken from her book, *The Hidden Truth of Cancer*,

> *'In 1964, only one person in 214 contracted cancer. Today it is one in three females and one in two males. The determining factor between health and disease is pH.'*

Secondly, I have had much success in my own practice using the methods I have set out in this chapter. To demonstrate this, I share a case study of one of my clients.

Terence made contact with me via e-mail after being recommended by another therapist. I arranged a call with him to ascertain what his health issues were. During the call Terence told me that he had been diagnosed with irritable bowel syndrome (IBS) and gout, both inflammatory conditions. Due to the fact that the gout was causing acute pain and swelling in his foot, Terence was struggling to work as a personal trainer. He also explained that due to the gout, he was finding driving difficult, and given we were over 40 miles apart, we decided to schedule a Skype call to carry out a full consultation. The only issue was that I did not have any availability for more than a week. As I did not want to leave Terence in discomfort I advised him to drink pure cherry juice daily until we spoke again. I had already experienced much success when recommending pure cherry juice to clients with gout and arthritis. A 2014 study by Northumbria University shows that drinking a concentrate made from tart Montmorency cherries, which possess anti-inflammatory and antioxidant properties, can help clear excess uric acid from the body in just a few hours. Gout is caused by defective metabolism of uric acid, which makes cherry juice a great supplement for sufferers to use. Dr Glynn Howatson from Northumbria University led the research and said,

'The study clearly shows that uric acid is lowered following consumption of the Montmorency cherry concentrate.'

A UK Gout Society spokesman acknowledged that Montmorency cherries could help reduce uric acid levels in the body but added,

'People with gout should go to their GP because it can be linked to other conditions such as stroke and psoriasis.'

Unfortunately for Terence, he had been using several different medications prescribed by his GP that were failing to bring sustainable relief of symptoms. Furthermore, because the medication prescribed included strong anti-inflammatory drugs, I was concerned about the long-term effects to his gut health. The gut is the first line of defense against illness and can be damaged by the use of non- steroid anti-inflammatory drugs (NSAIDs). You can read more on this subject in the Heal Your Gut chapter.

As planned, I spoke to Terence over Skype 10 days later and was pleased to hear he had experienced a significant reduction in his symptoms since using the juice. Together we proceeded to assess his diet and lifestyle to pinpoint anything that could be exacerbating his condition. It became apparent that although Terence did not have an unhealthy diet he did still have a number of inflammatory ingredients in his food that were likely contributing to his conditions. He was also not eating enough healthy fats, which are lubricating to joints. We decided to remove acid-forming foods, in particular dairy and gluten. Gluten is particularly significant, as many studies have noted that coeliac sufferers (with a hypersensitivity to gluten) experience joint pain and inflammation, which often progresses to arthritis, if coeliac is left undiagnosed for a considerable period. In his article called 'Cereal Grains, Humanity's Double Edged Sword', Dr. Loren Cordain of US Colorado State University describes how the gene code of gluten contains grains similar to human synovial tissue". Paul Chek, founder of the CHEK Institute, explains in his book *You Are What You Eat* how gluten often attacks synovial fluid around the joints, causing joint pain and arthritis. I put together a diet plan for Terence which included removing gluten and dairy, keeping sugar to an absolute minimum, continuing with the cherry juice, taking the supplements set out in the Heal Your Gut protocol and ensuring that he included plenty of anti-inflammatory foods into his diet alongside a healthy dose of omega-3 essential fatty acids. I provided Terence with the following anti-inflammatory food list and instructed him to ensure that he consumed a good selection on a daily basis, avoiding all inflammatory-causing foods, especially gluten. I arranged another Skype call to assess his progress for six weeks' time.

Anti Inflammatory Foods

- Wild Alaskan Salmon
- Fresh whole fruits
- Vegetables (dark green leafy are best)
- Green Tea
- Filtered Water
- Olive Oil
- Lean Poultry
- Nuts, legumes and seeds
- Spices (especially turmeric and ginger)

Inflammatory Foods

- Sugar
- Processed foods
- Fast foods
- Fried foods
- White bread
- Pasta
- Pasteurised dairy (especially ice cream)
- Hydrogenated Oils (such as vegetable and corn)
- Fizzy drinks
- Caffeine
- Alcohol

Six weeks later both Terence and I were delighted with the results. He told me he was pain-free, IBS-free, medication-free, back to work and had even lost weight, something that he had been trying to achieve for a while. I was also pleased that he had not found the plan restrictive, had plenty of choice and was enjoying this new way of eating. A great result for the anti-inflammatory approach and of course for Terence.

Whether inflammation is acute or chronic, we need to be grateful that our body is working to stimulate repair and healing. In the case of chronic, on-going inflammation it is imperative that we are able to notice the signs of impending inflammation so that we can take the necessary action to limit damage and reduce illness. Listen out for the messages your body is sending you instead of silencing them with medication. The body is persistent and the messages will be delivered more forcefully until appropriate improvements are made to diet and lifestyle. Never underestimate the power of your own body to self-heal when you provide it with the correct tools.

ACTION POINTS

- Look closely at your own diet to determine whether you eat enough anti-inflammatory foods

- Use the 'Get More' and 'Get Less' lists in this chapter to implement positive changes

- Think about the messages your body is sending you, and consider whether you are responding appropriately

- Add more foods rich in omega-3 to your diet in the form of nuts, seeds, avocado and oily fish

HEAL YOUR GUT

'All disease begins in the gut'
HIPPOCRATES

This chapter will help if you:

• Suffer from an auto-immune condition

• Have digestive issues or other symptoms of a food intolerance

• Have been over-exposed to a processed diet, medication or stress

As I say to my clients, the gut is the 'president' of the whole body. It has many crucial parts to play that govern how well the rest of your body is functioning. It is also the only organ that works independently to the brain. My personal experience of healing my own gut, which in turn healed my autoimmune condition, is testament to the vital role that the gut plays. I also see evidence in my clinic of the huge benefits of improving one's gut health.

In this chapter I explain the importance of good gut health, as well as taking you through my three-step gut healing protocol that you can hugely benefit from to maximise health and minimise symptoms.

Simply put, our gut is approximately nine metres of intestines starting at the mouth and ending at the anus. The primary function of the gut is digestion, controlled by the enteric nervous system, which some have called the 'second brain' due to the millions of neurons that reside there. However, if you have an unhealthy gut your body will let you know with far more than bloating, wind or diarrhoea. This is because the gut wall houses 70-80% of the cells that make up our immune system, so being consistently run down is a sign that you would benefit from improving your gut health. Another little-known gut function is the role it plays in our mental health and emotional wellbeing. Up to 90% of our body's serotonin is produced in the gastrointestinal tract. Serotonin is a chemical neurotransmitter that can affect mood, behaviour, appetite, digestion, sleep, memory and sexual desire and function. Research has found serotonin to be a chemical that balances mood, therefore a serotonin deficit leads to depression, yet another illness for which medication is prescribed without consideration as to the root cause.

It is most likely that you already have first-hand experience of the gut-brain connection. Have you had a 'gut wrenching' experience? Have you felt 'butterflies' through anxiety? Have you advised a friend to trust their 'gut instinct'? These are simple displays of gut-brain signals, which indicate just how intimately connected the gastrointestinal system and the brain are.

There is also a growing body of research into the links between the health of the gut and autism. The most recent research carried out by the US Arizona State University maintains that in nine out of ten cases, autistic people have common gut imbalances, such as a leaking gut, irritable bowel or fewer strains of good bacteria in the gut. This research is backed up by Dr Natasha Campbell McBride, the medical post-graduate and nutritionist who developed the well-known GAPS diet (Gut and Psychology Syndrome) a natural treatment for autism, ADHD, dyslexia, dyspraxia, depression and schizophrenia.

The 100 trillion bacteria that line your intestinal tract are approximately 3lbs or 2kgs in weight. This is an extremely complex living system that aggressively protects your body from outside offenders and is referred to as gut flora or microbiota. As it is impossible for our guts to remain completely sterile, the ideal ratio for gut bacteria is 85% good bacteria and 15% bad. Gut dysbiosis is the alteration of this balance and allows the bad bacteria to flourish. This condition is far more common than one would like to admit and is often undiagnosed, as it hides behind many other debilitating illnesses that take hold as a result of an unbalanced microbiota.

There are many signs and symptoms to show that you are suffering from an unhealthy gut, and among the most common are:

- Frequent wind and bloating
- Nausea
- Constipation/diarrhoea or both
- Headaches and migraines
- Fatigue and lethargy
- Sugar/refined carbohydrate cravings

Our gut bacteria is highly vulnerable to lifestyle and environmental factors. Unfortunately, because lifestyle and the environment have undergone huge changes in the last fifty years, our gut health has suffered. There has been a significant increase in auto-immune conditions, approaching epidemic proportions. A prime example of this is the rise of allergies, intolerances and related conditions such as coeliac disease, which have become far more prevalent in recent times. We now have a diet bombarded with artificial preservatives and additives that did not exist fifty years ago. In addition are environmental factors, such as worsening pollution and the introduction of genetically-modified foods, as recently as 1980, now heavily featured in our food chain. We are also more reliant on pharmaceutical medication to quick fix our health issues. I spoke to a client who was relying on daily ibuprofen tablets to keep headaches at bay but hadn't considered the fact that she was drinking little or no water, even though headaches are the number one sign of dehydration. Far too frequently we use medication to silence the important messages our body sends us.

Over time, processed food, alcohol, medication (counter or prescribed), stress and food intolerances will damage your gut lining and unbalance your gut flora. The most extreme cases can lead to intestinal permeability or leaky gut syndrome. This is a condition where the lining in the gut begins to wear away, creating holes big enough for food particles to pass through during digestion. Food passing through these holes will directly enter the bloodstream where the immune system thinks it is something that needs to be fought, prompting an autoimmune response.

The list of diseases being classified as autoimmune by the medical community is ever-growing. Please see the reference section at the back of this book for an up-to-date list. Some of the more prevalent conditions include:

- Lupus
- Scleroderma
- Diabetes
- Rheumatoid Arthritis
- Epstein-Barr Virus (EBV)
- Thyroid (Graves' Disease and Hashimoto's Disease)
- Multiple Sclerosis
- Psoriasis

If you have been diagnosed with an autoimmune condition it is likely that you have a degree of 'leaky gut' and will benefit from following the Heal Your Gut protocol. However, this protocol is not just for those who have received a diagnosis for a chronic illness. Due to the toxic onslaught we are now confronted with daily (read more about this in the chapter called Decrease Your Toxic Load), most people would experience health benefits after following this simple, three-step procedure to repair the gut lining and restore balance to the microbiota. For sustainable results, I recommend that this protocol be followed for a minimum of 12 weeks, followed by the implementation of diet and lifestyle changes.

STAGE 1 - REMOVE

The first stage of the Heal Your Gut process is to remove the foods that have been irritating and damaging the gut lining and disturbing the balance of the gut flora. The most definitive way to do this is by undergoing a food intolerance blood test, which will detect the foods that are creating an 'IGG antibody' reaction in your gut. Immunoglobulins or IGG are proteins made by the immune system to fight antigens such as bacteria, viruses and toxins. Symptoms that indicate you are having an IGG response to something you have inhaled, ingested or absorbed can vary greatly. Unlike an allergy, where a reaction is immediate, an IGG reaction is often much slower to take hold and can last from anywhere between an hour and three days. This delayed response can make offending foods difficult to identify without a test, and food intolerances are often misdiagnosed as other conditions.

Symptoms can be highly uncomfortable and at times debilitating, but as they are not considered life-threatening, a test is rarely available through the NHS. Many scientists and doctors believe that a food intolerance is not as significant as an allergy, as it does not prompt an immediate immune response. I believe this is a short-sighted viewpoint because food intolerances cause inflammation and chronic, constant inflammation is a precursor to disease.

Below is a non-exhaustive list of some of the most frequently occurring symptoms of food intolerances. Please see the reference section at the back of this book for a broader list:

- Acid Reflex
- Abdominal Pain/Cramps/Bloating
- Joint Pain/Arthritis
- Diarrhoea/Constipation
- Skin Issues (Eczema/Urticaria/Psoriasis/Acne)
- Sinus Issues (Sinusitis/Rhinitis)
- Headaches/Migraines

Without a food intolerance test, detection work is required to decipher the foods causing your symptoms. This is called an elimination diet, and requires methodically removing food types and noting any changes in symptoms. It can be extensive and time-consuming, which is far from ideal if you are experiencing a particularly immobilising symptom. When working with clients who are reluctant to take a food intolerance test, I recommend starting this first step by removing the top five ingredients in our diets which cause food intolerances – gluten, wheat, dairy, yeast and egg white.

These ingredients can cause acid and inflammation internally, which are precursors to disease; if you have an intolerance to them they will also be damaging the gut lining. However, there is no guarantee that these foods will be the cause of your specific intolerance. Working as a nutritionist, I have run tests on clients who have returned results with an intolerance to *broccoli*. This vegetable is a nutrient-dense super food but for those with sensitivity, it can act as a poison to the system over time. For anybody who wants to ensure that they are making the best nutrition choices to improve their health, an IGG antibody blood test is a powerful tool.

STAGE 2 - RESTORE

The second stage in the Heal Your Gut process is to seal any holes that may have appeared in the gut lining through the onset of intestinal permeability, or leaky gut syndrome. This happens when the epithelial junctions in the gut, which control what passes through the lining of the small intestine, allow substances to pass into the bloodstream. To heal and seal any damage to the gut lining, take heed of the ancient Greek physician, Hippocrates, when he said, 'Let food by thy medicine'.

Bone broth has gained popularity recently amongst the health conscious, however it is actually an ancient nourishing tradition. Bone broth is rich in minerals that support the immune system, and contains the healing compounds collagen, glutamine, glycine and proline. The collagen in particular heals your gut lining and reduces intestinal inflammation. This dish is simple to make but can be time-consuming, There are some good ready-made broths available in wholefood stores but fresh, homemade broth made with organic bones is far superior. Please see the reference section at the back of this book for my bone broth recipe.

If you are a vegetarian, or are struggling with the concept of bone broth it is still possible to heal and protect your gut lining through supplementation.

The most powerful ingredient in bone broth is collagen, the main supportive proteins that gives bone, cartilage and tendons their strength. Supplementing with collagen is a vital part of the gut healing process, particularly if you are not consuming bone broth.

Collagen also contains the amino acids proline and glycine, which are essential building blocks to repairing damaged intestinal lining.

L Glutamine is an essential amino acid and anti-inflammatory. This supplement repairs the gut and intestinal lining, as it fuels the cells that line the intestines and can help to repair a leaking gut. High levels of stress can also deplete your glutamine levels and leave you vulnerable to a leaky gut, which is yet another reason to supplement with L-glutamine. I recommend that both supplements are taken twice daily throughout the gut healing process.

STAGE 3 - REPLENISH

The final stage serves to rebalance the gut flora by replenishing the good bacteria in the gut that have likely been destroyed over time due to diet, medication and lifestyle. This can be done by including fermented, probiotic rich foods in your diet, such as live goats' milk kefir, sauerkraut and kimchi. Probiotics are the live, friendly bacteria and yeasts that are hugely beneficially to the digestive system.

As well as consuming probiotic rich foods, I also recommend introducing a daily probiotic supplement. Food and the pharmaceutical industry have changed so drastically in the last five decades that it has become almost impossible to sustain a healthy, balanced gut flora. I believe that a daily dose of probiotics is essential to maintain health and protect your gut. Choose your probiotic wisely, as there are many factors to consider. Unfortunately, almost all of the probiotic products sold in the supermarket are not of a high enough standard to survive the gastric juices in the gut, so they are not even reaching the location where they are most needed. Furthermore, they are often provided in yoghurt form, a highly concentrated dairy food, which is often the cause of food intolerance. The key factors to consider when choosing a probiotic are as follows:

- Brand – choose a trusted company who source high-quality ingredients
- Strains – look for multiple beneficial bacteria strains (see reference section for a comprehensive list)
- CFU – Colony-forming units are a measure of viable bacterial or fungal cells, and a high-quality supplement will have at least 15 billion.
- Variation – Do not stick to the same brand, as you will be consistently providing your body with the same strands of bacteria, which will create an imbalance over time. Regularly change the probiotic you use to ensure that you are exposed to a variation of strands.

The Heal Your Gut protocol needs to be followed, along with a healthy diet for a minimum of 12 weeks. By correctly identifying food intolerances, healing the gut lining and rebalancing the gut flora you will experience an improvement in digestive issues, irritable bowel and symptoms relating to auto-immune conditions. These improvements will be a direct result of a reduction in the inflammation occurring inside your body.

Once the gut lining has healed and the friendly bacteria are repopulated, you may be able to eat foods that previously you could not tolerate, with little or no reaction. However, if you would like to reintroduce foods that you have removed after the 12-week period, I recommend you seek advice from a nutritionist to ensure that you do not trigger any adverse reactions. Many of my clients implement bone broth or probiotics into their daily lives as a healthy habit to safeguard gut health and optimise wellness.

ACTION POINTS

- Identify and remove the foods you are intolerant to, either with an elimination diet or by undergoing a food intolerance blood test.

- Begin to heal your gut lining using the recommended supplements and/or with homemade bone broth, using the recipe in the reference section.

- Introduce a high-quality probiotic supplement to rebalance the friendly bacteria in your gut.

- Decide which of these health disciplines you will continue to use after the twelve-week period in order to protect your all-important gut health.

DECREASE YOUR TOXIC LOAD

*'If you don't recognise an ingredient,
your body won't either'*
KAREN SALMONSOHN

This chapter will help if you:

- Want to take control of what goes in and on your body

- Want to reduce your exposure to toxic chemicals but don't know where to start

- Want to take a holistic approach to health and healing

According to The Global Healing Centre it is not unusual for the average person to come into contact with 2.1 million toxins on a daily basis. Further research carried out by US University of California confirms these findings, documenting that the average person is exposed to cancerous levels of toxins in their lifetime. We will look at the ways in which we are regularly exposed to toxins and whether it would be beneficial for our health to decrease our toxic load.

The definition of a toxin in the Cambridge dictionary is, 'A poisonous substance that causes disease', I would argue that it is the dose that makes the poison. Unfortunately, in today's food and pharmaceutical industries we are often unknowingly exposed to significant doses of toxins that over time can be seen to have a poisonous effect on our bodies. We are experiencing a multitude of significant factors, which have led us into a global health epidemic. The way we produce food has changed more in the last 50 years than in the previous 10,000. In the 1940s, the use of synthetic herbicides and pesticides became widespread, which led to a myriad of toxic chemicals working their way into our soil and ultimately our food chain. The following decade saw the introduction of growth hormones and antibiotics being administered to farm animals. Although the EU banned the use of a variety of these hormones in farming in 1980, new trade deals with the US (where legislation is not in place) may mean that they may make it back on to our plates sometime soon. Then in the mid-90s, tomatoes became the first crop to be genetically engineered and grown commercially. Today, unless you are purchasing organic food it is likely that you are exposing yourself to genetically modified foods that have been grown though the use of synthetic pesticides. Furthermore, your meat may be laced with antibiotics, as figures from the Soil Association state that 40% of all antibiotics in the UK are given to farm animals. The overuse of antibiotics in farming is creating an army of superbugs such as E. -coli, and is the main reason that we have such high levels of resistance to these drugs now.

In addition to this, the use of artificial sweeteners, preservatives and additives have become commonplace, and fast food chains supplying cheap, processed food are far too readily available.

Although there is much research into the safety of these practices there is also mounting and conflicting evidence about the dangers. This makes it difficult for consumers to decipher the barrage and arrive at an educated decision. I believe that it is no coincidence that since we have begun to tamper so heavily with our food chain we have seen a dramatic increase in allergies and intolerances, as well as conditions such as diabetes, heart disease, cancer and Alzheimer's disease, to name just a few.

But it's not just our food chain that is responsible for our increasing levels of toxic exposure, as the products we use on our skin and to clean our home also make a huge contribution to the 2.1 million toxins that we are exposed to on a daily basis.

You may have heard yet more startling facts, including 60% of the chemicals in our cosmetics enter our bloodstream within 26 seconds of application. Before becoming anxious each time you moisturise, it is worth remembering that our skin is made up of several layers and does *not* act like a sponge, absorbing everything it comes in contact with. However, there is certainly evidence that some ingredients applied to our bodies can be transported into the bloodstream. In 1775, Percival Pott, an English surgeon, became the first person to demonstrate the link between environmental toxins and cancer, when he noticed an increase in scrotal cancer in chimney sweeps. He discovered this was due to skin contact with the polycyclic aromatic hydrocarbons present in soot. More recently, scientists have established that the hydrocarbons are in fact harmless, but certain enzymes in the skin convert them into reactive compounds that can damage DNA at a cellular level and cause cancer.

It would be almost impossible to put an exact figure on the speed and quantity of harmful chemicals absorbed because of the amount of variables between products and users. We are all unique and skin enzyme activity can vary greatly from person to person.

The skin is the body's largest detoxification organ and, along with the liver, kidney, lungs and large intestines, works continuously to eliminate toxins from our body. This is the reason that we often get skin complaints when we have a poor diet, and why heavy drinkers often have issues with the liver and smokers with the lungs. In my clinics and workshops, I advise my clients to take responsibility and ownership for their health by limiting toxin exposure. One of the most frequent questions I am asked is, 'Why do we need to worry about toxins; isn't that why we have detoxification organs?'

I explain that if we are living in and looking after a healthy body our detoxification organs are well-equipped to cope with the filtration of internal toxins and a proportion of external toxins.

Internal toxins are produced inside us; they are both created and fought by the body. Internal toxins include bad bacteria, viruses and waste from the process of cellular breakdown and renewal. Our metabolism and digestive system will also create internal toxins which will be eliminated using our detoxification organs.

External toxins are those we are exposed to outside the body but still need to be eliminated using our detoxification organs.

These include pollution, pesticides, cigarette smoke, alcohol and processed foods, as well as certain chemicals in skincare, hygiene and cleaning products. External toxins are far more difficult for the body to neutralise and excrete, and as a result are often stored in fat cells, leading to cellular damage. As previously established, external toxins are now far more prevalent than they were just 50 years ago, demonstrating that we are now facing an external toxin onslaught. This leaves our organs overworked and inflamed, depositing toxins inside our body instead of eliminating them. Toxins deposited in our body can lead to cysts, tumours, rheumatism, arthritis and cancer. US Stony Brook University in New York researched several cancers to determine how much risk was associated with environmental factors. They concluded that up to 90% of the most common cancers were caused by external toxins such as pollution and diet. These results highlight the importance of reducing your toxic load to preserve and protect your health.

Knowing where to start when you have decided to take a holistic approach to health by reducing exposure to harsh chemicals can be overwhelming. I have therefore compiled a list of the top five sources of toxins and how to reduce your exposure.

1. Processed food

The definition of processed food is any alteration of food from its natural state prior to eating, which can include cooking or freezing. While I appreciate the benefits of a raw vegan diet, this is far from realistic for many people. A more constructive approach to minimising processed food is to empower yourself with the knowledge of ingredients to minimise or avoid. In the chapter called Clean Eating Simplified, this subject is covered in more detail. When purchasing packaged food it is imperative to read the label, and never assume that all food is fit for human consumption just because it is on a supermarket shelf. You do not have to be a scientist, nutritionist or chef to realise that when a packaged item of food has a long list of incomprehensible ingredients, it has been highly processed. There is an ever-increasing list of ingredients to be aware of in processed food; a simple take on this is that if you don't recognise an ingredient, your body won't either.

In particular, white processed foods are to be minimised or avoided because of their highly-refined nature. White bread, white rice and pasta start life as whole grains but many minerals, vitamins and fibre are removed in an effort to extend their shelf life. Being empty of nutrients makes white grains easy to digest, creating spikes in blood sugar and insulin levels, which over time can contribute to Type 2 diabetes. By replacing processed white grains with whole grains, such as brown or wild rice, whole-wheat pasta, barley and oats, you will be decreasing your toxic load and stabilising your blood sugar levels.

One addition to most processed foods – sugar – is arguably the most toxic ingredient in the modern diet, due to the quantity in which it is used. There is a growing scientific consensus that added sugar can be just as toxic to the liver as alcohol. This topic is covered in full in the chapter called Reduce Your Sugar Fix.

2. Non-organic food

A common objection regarding organic produce is the fact that it is usually far more expensive than the non-organic alternative. There is a mounting body of evidence for the link between pesticides and many chronic conditions, as well as cancer, birth defects, reproductive disorders, Parkinson's disease, Alzheimer's, amyotrophic lateral sclerosis (ALS), diabetes, cardiovascular disease and chronic respiratory diseases. Organic food is therefore a worthwhile expense and one that we ought to be prioritising, above and beyond life's other luxuries. Are you putting a price on your health by ruling out organic food because of the cost?

The main reason organic food is often more costly is because organic certification is a long and arduous process for farmers. In the UK there are nine organic control bodies, none of which will approve organic certification until prohibited substances have not been used for a full 36 months. This makes the process hugely expensive for any farmer making the transition to organic. However, there are many farms who have not applied for, or been granted organic certification but do their best to harvest produce to organic standards. This means that they have a better standard of crops and meat, without the 'certified' price tag. It is worthwhile to research the farms and butchers in your local area as you may be able to source better produce without paying a premium.

I can fully appreciate the increased cost involved in becoming a totally organic shopper. Therefore, knowing where to substitute to benefit health is crucial. It is useful to refer to the Environmental

Working Group (EWG) 2016 Shoppers' Guide to Pesticides in Produce. The 'Clean Fifteen' shows a list of fruit and vegetables with the lowest levels of pesticides, and the 'Dirty Dozen', lists the fruits and vegetables with the highest levels of pesticides. The EWG compiled this data in the US, where there are significant differences to UK farming. However, The Expert Committee on Pesticide Residues published a UK equivalent last updated in September 2016, and the results are listed below, starting with those with the most to those with the least chemical residue:

The Dirty Dozen

- Apples
- Strawberries
- Grapes
- Celery
- Peaches
- Spinach
- Sweet Bell Peppers
- Nectarines
- Cucumbers
- Cherry Tomatoes
- Snap Peas
- Potatoes

The Clean Fifteen

- Avocados
- Sweet Corn*
- Pineapples
- Cabbage
- Sweet Peas
- Onions
- Asparagus
- Mangoes
- Papayas
- Kiwi
- Eggplant/Aubergine
- Grapefruit
- Cantaloupe/Melon
- Cauliflower
- Sweet potatoes

Corn is largely Genetically Modified Organism (GMO) in the UK, so opt for Organic where possible

3. Beauty, skincare and hygiene products

As previously discussed in this chapter, our daily toxic onslaught does not stop with food. It is just as important to be 'label savvy' with the products in your bathroom as it is in the kitchen. The industry regulations for beauty, skincare and hygiene products leave much to be desired, which means the consumer is left in a vulnerable position. Many of the ingredients that make it on to our skin and in some cases into our bloodstream are synthetic chemicals that can disrupt our endocrine system and are often known carcinogens.

Fear not, I don't relish the thought of only using coconut oil as an anti-ageing cream and going make up-free for the rest of my days. It's about compromise – assessing what products you use currently and making some improvements.

Below is a list of commonly used products with the average number of synthetic and potentially harmful chemicals lurking in each:

- Suncream – 9
- Toothpaste – 10
- Shampoo – 15
- Deodorant – 15
- Blusher – 16
- Fake Tan – 22
- Hair Dye – 22
- Eye Shadow – 26
- Body Lotion – 32
- Lipstick – 33

The good news is that there are many natural alternatives to these products now readily available in stores and online. I highly recommending using the free downloadable app for smart phones called Think Dirty. This app scores beauty products out of 10 according to the toxicity of the ingredients. Manufacturers are aware that the consumer is becoming more 'chemical conscious' and they therefore use clever packaging and wording to convince buyers that their product is 'natural'. Using the Think Dirty app will reveal the true quality of the ingredients, regardless of the enticing packaging.

Small changes can make a big difference with regards to toxic exposure. For example, if you were to choose just two products from the list that you are likely to use twice a day such as lipstick and body lotion. There are on average 65 synthetic chemicals in these products, giving a combined daily total of 130 when used twice daily. Multiplying 130 by the days of the year, 365, we arrive at a total of 47,450. This is the number of synthetic chemicals that you could decrease your exposure to each year simply by choosing a more natural alternative to just *two* regular beauty products.

To help you further, below is a list of the top five offending chemicals found in personal care products and their known side-effects:

1. Phthalates – Linked to breast cancer, early puberty in girls and obesity in children
2. Parabens – Present in 75-95% of cosmetics and have been found in biopsies of breast tumours
3. Ethylene Oxide – Linked to an increased risk of breast cancer
4. Lead – Proven to reduce fertility; ongoing research into its links to learning disabilities and behavioural problems
5. Triclosan – Classified as a pesticide, seriously disrupts hormones, in particular thyroid

4. Household Cleaning Products

Household cleaning products are a more obvious exposure to toxins, not least because of the chemical hazard symbol featured on most packaging. Many consumers of these products will refuse to use them without the protection of rubber gloves, yet several of the chemicals are identical to those used in beauty, skincare and hygiene products. For example, sodium lauryl/laureth sulphate (SLS) is a widely used ingredient in many cleaning products, including washing up liquid, laundry powder, carpet cleaners, toilet cleaners and all-purpose cleaners. However, it can also be found in most brands of shampoo, toothpaste and face wash, to name a few. *The Journal of the American College of Toxicology* published a report entitled 'The Safety Assessment of Sodium Lauryl Sulfate and Ammonium Lauryl Sulfate' and stated that SLS has 'a degenerative effect on the cell membranes because of its protein denaturing properties'. The author adds, 'high levels of skin penetration may occur even at low use concentration.'

Although we are not purposefully ingesting these products, we are often touching them and using them to sanitise surfaces where food may be prepared.

On average, there are in excess of 150 toxic substances linked to cancer that are regularly being used in our homes in chemical cleaning products. The testing of these products is far from sufficient, with less than 20% being tested for the effects on our health and not even 1% for chronic damage to health. Perhaps most frightening of all, women in the cleaning profession who work alongside toxic cleaning products have a 55% higher risk of developing cancer than women outside of this industry.

Just as with beauty, skincare and hygiene products, there are more natural brands of cleaning products readily available to purchase. You can also try making your own, which is not only far more cost-efficient, it is easy too. For example, lemon juice is a natural bleach, white vinegar is an excellent glass cleaner and baking soda has multiple uses, including deep cleaning toilets and ovens. (See the reference section for my favourite DIY cleaning product recipes).

5. Toxic People

Perhaps the easiest way to reduce your toxic load with immediate effect is to limit your exposure to toxic people. We have all come across a person who has disregarded our feelings, made us feel insignificant and ploughed through our boundaries. Each relationship we have is individual and often complex, and sometimes we may not identify a relationship as toxic because it didn't start out that way, instead it slowly turned sour. Other times a relationship may not be consistently toxic and instead behaviour that makes you feel drained or worthless is periodically displayed. Toxic people may come in the form of friends, colleagues, partners or family and often we feel that the type of relationship we have with them dictates how we manage the toxicity. Best-selling author and playwright Dee Dee M Scott says:

'Toxic people are like cancer, if you keep them in your
life they will destroy your dreams, hopes and ambitions.'

If you have a particular person in your life who consistently makes you feel manipulated, judged, confused, unsupported, drained, worthless or negative then it is imperative you take steps to manage the relationship so that it is no longer damaging to you. If you feel the situation is unmanageable then you are left with little choice but to remove them from your life. Whether it is a colleague or partner, toxic relationships must end for your own health. Studies have shown the long-lasting effects of stress on the brain, and negative emotions triggered by toxic people will create a stress response. Learning to handle toxic people is self-preservation. My top five tips for dealing with toxic people are:

1. Show empathy and compassion towards the person, but ensure that self-compassion takes priority.
2. Be the behaviour that you want to see. Not only are you rising above them, you are demonstrating your expectations.
3. Limit the time you spend in their company by removing yourself from any situation you find uncomfortable, or get good at suddenly changing the subject during your conversations.
4. Find your positive posse and spend more time in their company. This will raise your vibration and highlight how toxic other relationships are.
5. Do not feel guilty if you have to let them go from your life. This is not an act of cruelty; it is an act of self-love.

Decreasing your toxic load is not about overhauling your entire life in one go. Instead, focus on making one small change at a time that will eventually become one big, healthy transformation.

ACTION POINTS

- Become aware of food labels so you are able to avoid toxic ingredients and make better choices

- Decide which beauty, skincare and hygiene products you would like to change first and seek a more natural alternative

- Have a go at making your own cheap and natural cleaning products, using the recipes in the reference section

- Take it a step at a time. Decrease your toxins by taking one small step at a time to minimise your risk of illness

CHANGE YOUR SUGAR FIX

'The deadliest poisons in the world taste sweet'
NENIA CAMPBELL

This chapter will help if you:

- Are caught in a perpetual sugar cycle and need help to break it

- Want to know the difference between sugar and artificial sweeteners

- Want to know the real reason you can't just have one chocolate – it has nothing to do with will power

Once upon a time, fat was public health enemy number one. Slowly but surely the nation is waking up to the fact that the real enemy is actually sugar and most of us are already addicted.

Recent research conducted by Public Health England revealed that UK families are consuming as much as 483g or 120 teaspoons of sugar a day, which accounts for more than half their daily calorie intake.

Sugar comes in many forms, often cleverly disguised by a multitude of names, such as sucrose, fructose, dextrose, lactose, sorbitol, xylitol, stevia, aspartame and syrup.

Sucrose is a naturally occurring saccharide found in many plants. It is made up of fructose, which is fruit sugar and dextrose, also known as glucose. Dextrose is the main component of starch and is quickly absorbed by the body; hence its use in energy drinks. You may have also heard of lactose, which is the sugar found in milk, and high fructose corn syrup, a highly processed sugar found in packaged foods. Xylitol, sorbitol and stevia are used as alternative sweeteners alongside aspartame, a controversial artificial sweetener.

We will take a closer look at sugar consumption as well as how sugar impacts our body, and why the food industry is determined to overload us with it regardless of the impact on our health.

In 1950, the American Scientist Ancel Keys conducted mass research into the links between diet and cardiovascular disease. His findings shaped the dietary advice given by healthcare professionals for the coming decades. Keys concluded that a diet rich in saturated fats would lead to coronary heart disease. This study also secured low fat and no fat food brands a place on every supermarket shelf and the store cupboard staple of the health conscious, sending the world into the grasps of fat phobia. Fat was demonised, which meant that the real culprit went under the radar, while cardiovascular disease continued to rise.

An American Endocrinologist named Robert Lustig, in a 90-minute lecture he recorded in 2009 for The University of California called 'Sugar: The Bitter Truth', finally revealed the truth and it went viral on the internet. Lustig argues that fructose can be consumed safely within whole fruits and vegetables because they contain fibre. But he maintains that the liver is damaged by added sugar in food and beverages, particularly convenience food and soft drinks. Lustig's research examines links between excess consumption of fructose and the development of metabolic syndrome, which can include Type 2 diabetes, high blood pressure, cardiovascular disease, non-alcoholic fatty liver disease and obesity.

Fructose is exclusively metabolised by the liver, and our liver can only store about 60-90g of sugar at any one time. Beyond 90g the liver detects more fructose than can be used by the body for energy. That excess fructose is broken down by the liver and transformed into fat globules called triglycerides, some of which are exported into the bloodstream and deposited around your midsection and internal organs. To put the 90g of sugar that the liver can store into perspective, there are about 35g of sugar in a 330ml can of cola. Many popular brands of cereal contain 9-10g, or more than 2 teaspoons, of sugar per serving, and a chocolate milkshake may contain a shocking 48g of sugar, which amounts to 12 teaspoons. According to research carried out for Jamie Oliver's 2015 *Sugar Rush* documentary, it is now very apparent that the average Briton is consuming 160g of sugar daily. Further research carried out by Public Health England (PHE) in 2016, as part of the Change4Life campaign, found that children in England consume more than 11g of sugar at breakfast time alone. This equates to eating three sugar cubes, more than half of daily recommendations for children. The recommended daily maximum is no more than 20g or five cubes of sugar for four-to-six-year-olds and no more than 24g or six cubes for seven-to-ten-year-olds per day. The PHE survey concluded that by the end of each day children would have consumed more than three times the recommendations. As a nutritionist and a parent, I find these figures alarming, not least because they confirm that one of our body's detoxification organs faces a toxic overload of sugar on a daily basis. Furthermore, mounting evidence is identifying sugar as the cause behind many modern-day health epidemics, such as diabetes, heart disease and obesity. NHS guidelines state that added sugars should not make up more than 5% of daily calorie intake from food and drink. This is about 30g of sugar or seven teaspoons a day for those aged eleven and over. In essence, our National Health Service advises us to have less sugar daily than is added to one single can of fizzy cola.

It is evident that there is insufficient legislation in the UK regarding sugar usage in food and beverages, which leaves the onus on consumers to educate themselves. Limited legislation on sugar use has led to a huge increase in consumption. Last century the average consumption was only 2kg per person per year, but due to the increased use in packaged foods sugar consumption is now over 1kg per person per week, and all the while obesity, diabetes and cardiovascular disease are spiralling out of control. Who is to blame? Do consumers lack willpower or do manufacturers lack ethics?

Every brand in the food industry will invest vast amounts of money each year in researching and developing the bliss point in their products. The bliss point is a term coined by American market researcher and psychophysicist, Howard Moskowitz, known for his pioneering work in product optimisation. The bliss point is the perfect amount of sugar, salt and fat used to optimise palatability. Moskowitz describes the bliss point as 'that sensory profile where you like food the most'.

Paul Stitt, author of *Beating the Food Giants*, has first-hand experience of the many tricks the food industry will use to keep you reaching for more, as he worked for many years as a research scientist for Quaker. Stitt says,

'Many nasty tricks are used by Food Giants to make you overeat. Adding lots of fat, sugar and salt are obvious ones.'

Pringles are synonymous with their 'once you pop, you can't stop' slogan and I'm sure you have blamed your willpower more than once on your inability to quit after just one chocolate. In actual fact, willpower has very little to do with reducing fat, sugar and salt when we consider the tricks that food giants are using to openly pedal these modern-day 'drugs'. Obviously there are other contributing factors to the surge in illness and obesity, such as personal responsibility and lifestyle. However, it is truly frightening what lengths and expense the food industry goes to, to make a product so irresistible, so tasty, so perfectly engineered to get us to not just like them, but to want more and more of them.

The neural centre in the brain that regulates appetite is the hypothalamus. This is often referred to as the 'appestat' as it behaves like a thermostat for your appetite. Scientists and endocrinologists have come to realise that because fructose is mainly handled by the liver, very little reaches the brain, so the appetite remains active regardless of intake. Refined sugar, salt and fat numb the appestat. It is only when we eat the correct balance of nutrients that we experience satiety, signalled by the brain. Therefore, by consuming foods high in refined sugar and low in fats and proteins we are setting ourselves up for cravings and binging. What's worse, the food giants know this and they use it to drive profits with little regard for consumers' health.

Dr Norman Joliffe of US Columbia University's School of Public Health wrote in his study on how to reset your appestat and reduce hunger:

> *'Infants do not have the natural ability to overeat.*
> *Overeating is a learned behaviour that needs to be*
> *unlearned to reduce hunger.'*

Excess sugar consumption has also been repeatedly shown to elevate dopamine levels, which control the brain's reward and pleasure centres, making it as addictive as many illegal drugs. Long-term consumption can lead to a reduction in dopamine levels, meaning a higher dose of sugar is required to achieve the same level of reward. High sugar consumption and binge eating may also instigate neurological and psychological consequences affecting mood and motivation.

According to research by Dr David Ludwig MD PhD, the part

of the brain that lights up when eating high sugar foods is the same part of the brain that's triggered by cocaine or heroin. It is clear to see that sugar is a drug, we are a nation of addicts and the food giants are the supplier. The huge price that we are paying for the perpetual sugar cycle we are in is our wellbeing, with an ever-increasing list of health issues that can be traced back to sugar:

- Increased risk of obesity, diabetes and heart disease
- Impaired immune function
- Chromium deficiency – a trace mineral that regulates blood sugar
- Accelerated ageing
- Tooth decay and gum disease
- Behaviour and cognition in children
- Increase release of stress hormones, such as adrenaline, epinephrine and cortisol

It is clear to see that insulin resistance from excess sugar consumption is damaging to the body in many ways. However, the most controversial and provocative of the implications of this hypothesis is that sugar may cause or exacerbate cancer.

Gary Taubes, the Harvard graduate and award-winning science writer who specialises in diet and nutrition, explains the link between increased insulin levels and a greater chance of developing cancer in his book '*The Case Against Sugar*'

> *'But why should cancer, which happens when*
> *cells grow out of control, be affected by high*
> *levels of insulin? It's because insulin does many*
> *things in the human body, including stimulating*
> *cells to multiply and tumours to grow.'*

Sugar feeds tumours and encourages cancer growth. The fact that cancer cells uptake sugar at 10-12 times the rate of healthy cells is the basis of Position Emission Tomography (PET) scans, which is one of the most accurate pieces of equipment for detecting cancer. PET scans use radioactive glucose to detect cancerous cells, and when patients drink the sugar water it gets absorbed into any cancerous cells. Cancerous growths are highlighted because of the rate they absorb the glucose. Furthermore, in 1931 Nobel prize winner for medicine Otto Warburg discovered that cancer cells metabolise energy differently to healthy cells. He found that malignant tumours exhibit increased glycolysis, a process where glucose is used as fuel.

The link between sugar and cancer is not yet a concept that has been embraced by many oncologists or cancer charities.

Indeed, cancer charities often raise funds through coffee mornings and cake sales, which involve participants baking and selling cakes to raise funds for the charity. I often catch myself wondering if the nation would be so accepting if a cigarette brand offered to donate a percentage of their profits to cancer research. Other comparisons between the tobacco and sugar industries are difficult to ignore and highly disturbing. Sugar is the new tobacco, and in my opinion it is far worse because, unlike tobacco, it is being specifically marketed at children, with brightly-coloured packaging and cartoon character branding. It took 50 years before the link between smoking and lung cancer was acknowledged in the *British Medical Journal*, and the government introduced effective regulations. The tobacco industry vigorously defended its practices by planting doubt and confusion amongst the public and by buying the loyalty of scientists. Research carried out in 1967 by McGandy et al was discredited in 2016 in the *Journal of the American Medical Association (JAMA)*, claiming the sugar industry paid three highly influential Harvard scientists to discredit sugar's role in heart disease and shift the blame to fat once again. In 2015, an article by Anahad O'Connor published in the *New York Times* suggested that the Coca-Cola Company paid millions of dollars to fund research that blamed lack of exercise as the main factor in obesity and not the role of sugar.

The Cancer Research website has an article entitled '10 Persistent Cancer Myths Debunked' and myth number four is that cancer has a sweet tooth. The article states, 'While it's very sensible to limit sugary foods as part of an overall healthy diet and to avoid putting on weight, that's a far cry from saying that sugary foods specifically feed cancer cells.' I question whether this is the belief of Cancer Research UK or just another example of the sugar industry ensuring that their links to cancer are played down.

Dr Patrick Quillin PHD, RD, CNS, former Director of Nutrition for Cancer Treatment Center of America wrote in *Nutrition*

Science News in April 2000, 'It puzzles me why the simple concept "sugar feeds cancer" can be so dramatically overlooked as part of a comprehensive cancer treatment plan.' He went on to list five reasons why sugar and cancer are best friends. The full article can be found by visiting http://beatcancer.org/blog-posts/5-reasons-cancer-and-sugar-are-best-friends/ . It is a must read for anyone wanting to overcome or avoid cancer – just about all of us.

With mounting evidence on the adverse effects of sugar and the huge amounts of sugar being added to our food, how can we beat the food giants and avoid sugar addiction and disease?

On the Global Diabetes Community website, diabetes.co.uk, it states that sugar needs to be kept to a minimum, and recommends that one way of doing this is to use sweeteners. The suggestion is that sweeteners do not raise blood glucose levels, and unlike sugar, are calorie-free. Unfortunately, most sweeteners, with the exception of sugar alcohols and stevia, are man-made chemicals not found in nature. The human body was not designed to process these chemicals, which means that we are unable to absorb them, leading to gas, bloating and in some cases diarrhoea. Research has also shown that the appestat reacts the same way to sweeteners as it does to sugar, which can lead to increased desire, over-eating and weight gain. However, wind and weight gain are the least concerning side effects with regards to artificial sweeteners. Aspartame is the most commonly used sweetener and is also the most controversial. Aspartame is listed on the Food and Drug Agency's (FDA) 'generally regarded as safe' list (GRAS) with 75% of adverse reactions reported to the FDA linked to this sweetener, including heart palpitations, hyperactivity and thyroid dysfunction. In 1980 the FDA banned it after three independent scientists linked it to inducing brain tumours. However, in 1981, due to a change in government, the FDA re-approved aspartame for use once more. Then in 1983, despite much independent research into the detrimental effects, it was approved by the FDA for use in soft drinks. Today aspartame is present in most diet drinks, including the 'no added sugar' versions of juice, aimed at health-conscious parents. There are more than 900 published and peer-reviewed studies on the dangerous side effects of aspartame. The longest study was run for 22 years by Harvard University and concluded that just one drink per day containing aspartame led to a multiplied risk of blood cancer – leukaemia. I could write an entire book about aspartame but that has already been done. I would highly recommend reading *Sweet Poison* by Janet Starr Hall for a more in-depth literacy on the neurotoxin named aspartame.

As briefly mentioned, there are natural alternatives to sugar readily available that can be added to homemade dishes to satisfy any sweet tooth. The best way to beat the food giants is to make your food yourself, safe in the knowledge that the contents have not been chemically enhanced or artificially flavoured to alter the chemistry in your brain and ultimately lead you to overeating and ill health. I take a more in depth look at choosing fresh, wholesome ingredients to prepare your meals in the next chapter.

Healthier and more natural alternatives to refined or artificial sugar are listed below:

- Coconut Sugar (in moderation)
- Honey (in moderation)
- Blackstrap Molasses – unrefined sugar cane
- Naturally Occurring – as in fruit
- Dates – baking/snacking
- Sweet spices – eg: anise and cinnamon

It is also possible to reduce your added sugar consumption significantly by making simple food swaps. The swaps listed below will increase energy levels in comparison to the alternative and will also keep blood sugar levels stable and cravings at bay.

- Porridge oats with cinnamon or honey instead of sugary shop-bought cereals
- Sweet potatoes instead of white (starchy) potatoes
- Wholemeal bread/pasta instead of white bread/pasta
- Lean protein such as chicken or fish instead of burgers/pizza
- Homemade smoothies instead of shop-bought milkshakes
- Hummus and guacamole instead of sugary dips/sauces like ketchup
- Fruit, nuts or homemade treats instead of cakes and puddings

If you eat a Western diet it is highly likely you are eating way too much sugar, and you may or may not realise this. If you are aware, you have probably blamed your willpower but now realise you are merely the victim of the food giants who invest vast resources and funds into researching how they can turn their consumer into an addict. Being empowered with the knowledge of this, along with the information to implement better choices, you will now be able to break out of the perpetual sugar cycle that is far too common in today's society.

ACTION POINTS

- Release the shackles of the food industry giants by boycotting their processed products

- Monitor your family's daily sugar intake to ensure you are not over the recommended amount

- Check labels for sugar content. You will be surprised where sugar is added – even to bread

- Experiment at home with natural sugars. Make homemade no-added sugar, healthy alternatives to shop bought favourites

CLEAN EATING SIMPLIFIED

*'The food you eat can be the safest and most powerful
form of medicine or the slowest form of poison'*
ANN WIGMORE

This chapter will help if you:

- Are confused by the concept of 'clean eating'

- Want to know the difference between a good and
  bad protein, fat and carbohydrate

- Want to understand the hype around gluten-free
  and dairy free diets

These days, the term 'clean eating' is overused and frequently
misused. I have never particularly liked this phrase, first coined
by the media in the late nineties. While the term was created with
good intentions, the use of the word 'clean' has overtones that
suggest that if you aren't eating this way you are 'dirty'.

It also does not go far enough to describe what 'clean eating'
actually means, with the result that many believe that 'clean
eating' means an organic diet free from multiple food groups,
such as gluten, wheat, dairy and sugar. Although this may be how

it is sometimes portrayed, this is not my understanding of eating clean and most definitely not the advice I pass on to clients.

Clean eating is actually simple to follow and can optimise your health without over-complicating your fridge.

As I have mentioned, I often tell my clients that unless a food has 'walked, swam grew or flew, don't eat it'. This is clean eating in a nutshell. In my opinion, eating clean is using food *as* ingredients as opposed to using food *with* ingredients. The closer a food is to its natural state and the fewer additions it has received on its journey to your plate, the cleaner it is. Eating whole, real foods such as fruit, vegetables, whole grains, protein from both animal and plants, nuts, seeds and unrefined oils, minimally processed and packaged is the essence of the clean eating concept.

It is unrealistic to assume that clean eating has the same starting point for each person. Clean eating as a lifestyle is a staged journey. When I work alongside my clients to help them implement better eating habits we start by looking at how they are currently eating before deciding what needs to be reduced or replaced in their diet for better health.

It would be highly unrealistic to suggest to a busy mother who is currently using processed freezer meals that she must start to shop and eat completely organic food from the moment the consultation is over. In Decrease Your Toxic Load, I have documented the many benefits of organic food, however, this example is a journey of many miles best undertaken slowly and steadily for long-term results.

When studying at the CHEK institute I was taught to respect the 'rainbow bridge' journey of each individual. This journey is made with small, consistent and sustainable changes towards your goal. This approach is in opposition to sudden and abrupt modifications to a diet, which more often than not lead to poor results. I love explaining the rainbow bridge to my clients because their goal becomes instantly more achievable when broken down in this way.

Founder of the CHEK institute, Paul Chek writes,

> *'Through a lot of study and work, I've found that if we create what I refer to as a rainbow bridge, changes are more sustainable, without guilt, shame and blame being an issue.'*

Perhaps the most sensible place to begin your journey across the clean-eating rainbow bridge is to look at how close your diet is to Mother Nature. Understanding the traceability of your food is an integral part of healthy, clean eating. Eric Schlosser states in his 2001 book, *Fast Food Nation*,

> *'The food we have available to us today has changed more in the past 40 years than in the previous 40,000.'*

This is a huge issue because our bodies have not adapted at the same rate, making food far less bio available to us. Our bodies can struggle to recognise and utilise the food we are using for fuel. As Sally Fallon, founder of the Weston A Price Foundation, points out in her book *Nourishing Traditions*, as a nation we have never eaten so badly and never been so poorly. She says,

143

'Although heart disease and cancer were rare at the turn of the century, they now strike with increasing frequency, in spite of billions of dollars in research. One person in three dies of cancer, one in three suffers from allergies, one in ten will have ulcers and one in five is mentally ill.'

	GOOD	**BAD**
PROTEIN	Organic eggs, meat, fish, poultry and pulses	Processed meats such as salami and bacon, whey and soy
CARBOHYDRATES	Sweet potatoes, quinoa, brown rice, lentils, chickpeas, buckwheat, oats	Bleached white flour, rice and pasta, refined sugars, commercial cereals (even fortified ones)
FATS	Grass-fed butter, flaxseed, coconut oil, nuts, oily fish (salmon, trout, mackerel), avocado, oil olive *	Highly processed vegetable oils, margarine, anything labelled 'low-fat', fried food

olive oil has a low burning point and should therefore not be heated as the oil can turn rancid and create free radicals

It is evident that we need to take our diet back to basics and embrace the nourishing traditions Sally Fallon refers to by becoming label savvy and boycotting the abundance of processed foods that line our supermarket aisles. Suggesting to clients that they 'become label savvy' usually injects them with fear as they do not want to have to gain a degree in science to complete their weekly food shop. To simplify this process, use the table above which demonstrates non-exhaustive good and bad choices of the three macronutrients (protein, carbohydrates and fats) to make selecting food closer to nature far easier.

PROTEIN

Arguably the most important macronutrient of the three, protein is the building block of all of our cells. As the table demonstrates, good protein choices are traceable to a farm and do not come with a list of unrecognisable ingredients, unlike the proteins listed on the other side of the table. Organic is the best option, but remember the rainbow bridge, and if organic is an initial step too far then opting for a good source of protein as opposed to a processed version is a step in the right direction of clean eating. Bad proteins are highly processed and come in packets with multiple ingredients that are used to preserve and flavour the goods. Many of the ingredients listed will not be recognisable to our body, which will result in difficulty digesting, absorbing and using any of the limited nutrients that these products provide. I have also included soy and whey on the bad side of protein.

Both soy and soya are phytoestrogens and will weakly mimic oestrogen in our bodies, which has caused concern regarding the balance of hormones. However, the most alarming thing about soy is the fact that 81% of the global soybean crop is genetically modified, making it difficult for the body to recognise and utilise. Become label savvy to minimise or avoid. Soy is used in many 'health' foods as a protein source.

Whey is a by-product of dairy, and is the liquid remaining after milk has been curdled and strained. I will come to dairy shortly.

CARBOHYDRATES

These are our main source of energy and provide important nutrients found in fruits, grains and vegetables. They are made of fibre, starch and sugars. All the carbohydrates we eat and drink are broken down into glucose. The type, and amount you consume can make a difference to your blood glucose levels. The carbohydrates shown in the table as 'good' are a selection of complex carbohydrates. Fibre and starch are the two types of complex carbohydrates. Fibre is especially important because it promotes bowel regularity and helps to control cholesterol levels. Complex carbohydrates have more nutrients because they are higher in fibre and digest slower. They also provide slow release energy, longer satiety and stabilise blood sugar levels, making them a great option for weight control and diabetes management.

The carbohydrates on the bad side of the table are a selection of simple carbs, which comprise predominantly of added sugars. Our bodies metabolise simple carbs very quickly, raising blood sugar and energy levels fast, then bringing them crashing back down, initiating further sugar cravings and hunger, and so the perpetual sugar cycle begins (more on this in the Reduce Your Sugar Fix chapter). Simple carbohydrates are refined, processed, packaged, full of sugar and not part of a clean eating plan. When considering the rainbow bridge method, it is easy to make simple swaps from white foods to brown foods (bread, rice, pasta) as an initial step towards clean eating.

FAT

This macronutrient has been falsely accused of multiple crimes to health, making it a long-term enemy to the weight- and health-conscious. The low fat diet industry first began in 1840, so with nearly 200 years of low-fat diets, why are we as a nation fatter than ever? The fats shown in the table as 'good' are unsaturated fat, polyunsaturated and monounsaturated. Essential fatty acids (EFAs) are polyunsaturated. Only two fatty acids are known to be essential for humans – alpha-linolenic acid (an omega-3 fatty acid) and linoleic acid (an omega-6 fatty acid). The shocking truth about fats is that essential fatty acids (EFAs) actually *increase* the rate at which body fat burns and *decrease* body fat production. It's a win-win situation.

This is explained fully in the excellent book *Fats that Heal and Fats that Kill* by Dr Udo Erasmus. I would recommend this book to anyone who has been brainwashed by the dangerous low-fat, no-fat diet industry that will inevitably make you ill in the long term. Dr Udo Erasmus discusses the many benefits of consuming EFAs. The one fat fact that usually makes my clients sit up and take note is that good fat will reduce the body fat you are carrying, particularly around the abdomen and waist, which is usually most people's trouble spot. James Duigan is a personal trainer renowned for keeping the likes of Elle Macpherson and Rosie Huntington-Whiteley in perfect shape and health. In his book *The Clean and Lean Diet,* he says;

> *'Good fats make you skinny. Having a quality*
> *Omega-3 oil everyday burns fat around your middle,*
> *reduces inflammation throughout your entire body*
> *and can reduce sugar cravings.'*

In contrast, the fats shown in the table as 'bad' are the fats to avoid. These are the toxic fats that are associated with heart disease, hardening of the arteries, cellulite and obesity. This is the fat that will promote cancer, make us more susceptible to heart disease and stroke and slow you down as opposed to give you energy. So where do we find these bad fats lurking? Unfortunately, this type of fat is found in many foods, particularly if you are eating a highly processed diet, and they are known as 'trans' fats. Trans fats are used extensively in frying, baked goods, biscuits, icings, crisps, packaged snack foods, microwave popcorn, and some margarine. Margarine (and other low fat spreads) is a completely processed product, one molecule away from being plastic; its real colour is grey – a yellow dye is added to make it look more like butter. Incidentally, it was invented at the same time as the diet industry. Research has shown that even small amounts of artificial trans fats can increase the risk for heart disease by increasing LDL 'bad' cholesterol and decreasing HDL 'good' cholesterol. The best way to keep on top of the fats in your diet is to eat clean. It is very hard for bad fats to sneak into your diet when you are preparing your own meals instead of relying on packets. Eating clean does not have to be a time-consuming chore. It is just as easy to grill a piece of salmon while you boil some quinoa and put a handful of leafy green vegetables and avocado on your plate as it is to put some nutrient-deficient frozen chips and chicken kiev into the oven. The most effortless way to step foot on that rainbow bridge and begin your clean eating journey is to replace anything that you are currently consuming from the bad side of the table with a better alternative from the good side. If you find this concept too overwhelming, try not to change everything at once. Simply choose three things from the bad side that you regularly consume and swap them for a better alternative. Once the better alternatives are store cupboard staples you can then move on to the next three changes. Slowly but surely you will make your way across that rainbow bridge and be rewarded with health and vitality as you go.

To help you understand better alternatives, I have listed some other everyday food swaps in the Reduce Your Sugar Fix chapter that are easy to do but can make a big impact on your health and waistline.

The definition of clean eating is often misconstrued and instead of focusing on whole, natural, unprocessed foods many believe it is necessary to become gluten- and dairy-free in order to completely embrace the clean eating way. Although I believe there are many benefits in reducing these food groups, it is not necessary to eradicate them entirely.

Gluten is a protein in wheat, but it is also found in rye and barley too. Oats can contain gluten because they are harvested on the same equipment as gluten grains. Gluten-free diets were once reserved for those who suffer from coeliac disease or gluten sensitivity. However, it has now become popular to 'go gluten-free' after benefits such as weight loss and increased energy have been heavily reported in the media. This trend has led to an increase in the availability of gluten-free produce in supermarkets and restaurants as manufacturers accommodate the demand. The general consensus among doctors and dieticians is that avoiding gluten is pointless unless you suffer with a digestive condition that does not tolerate it. Dr. Daniel Leffer, assistant professor of medicine at Harvard Medical School states,

> *'People who are sensitive to gluten may feel better,*
> *but a larger portion will derive no significant benefit*
> *from the practice of eliminating gluten.'*

Since no significant research has been funded or completed on the benefits of a gluten-free diet, mainstream medical professionals have disregarded it. Like many holistic practitioners and functional medicine doctors, I have witnessed huge improvements in clients who have reduced, or eliminated gluten from their diet. What's more, I am yet to hear a valid argument as to why we need it, and have not yet come across a person who has a severe gluten deficiency.

Doctor Alessio Fasano, the director of the Center for Coeliac Research and Treatment, and Chief of Pediatric Gastroenterology and Nutrition at the Massachusetts General Hospital for Children, published a ground-breaking study in the *Annals of Medicine* in 2003 that established the prevalence rate of coeliac disease at one in 133 in the USA. He says,

> *'Prevalence is rising and we're in the midst of an epidemic. Based on our study it seems the diagnosis has doubled every 15 years in North America. Why? I think it goes back to the microbiome. There are antibiotics, our diet has changed, we travel more. There have been so many changes in the past 50 years.'*

Since the agricultural revolution, gluten has become a staple part of the modern diet, appearing with alarming regularity. Popular books such as *Grain Brain* by Dr David P Permultter and *Wheat Belly* by Dr William Davis argue that our bodies weren't designed to cope with gluten, particularly in the amounts it is now being eaten. Furthermore, gluten is a frequent ingredient in many of the processed foods that we are warned to avoid when eating clean, such as bread, cakes, biscuits and sauces. Gluten is an ingredient that can cause inflammation, the precursor to disease. Dr Alessio Fasano tell us,

> *'We don't digest gluten completely, which is unlike
> any other protein. The immune system seems to see
> gluten as a component of bacteria and deploys
> weapons to attack it, and creates some collateral
> damage we call inflammation.'*

When working with clients, I suggest that gluten is at least minimised in the diet, as I believe in the benefits of a clean, unprocessed diet. I especially make this recommendation if the client has been diagnosed with an inflammatory condition or it is evident that they are suffering from inflammation throughout the body. A prime example is when clients have arthritis, an inflammatory condition that has been linked to gluten because the gene code of gluten is remarkably similar to that of synovial fluid, the fluid around our joints. Also, gluten is one of the top five foods which are detected in food intolerance blood tests, and on this evidence alone I believe it is highly valuable for overall health for us to limit the consumption of gluten in our modern diet.

Dairy has a similar story to gluten, whereby it has become fashionable to be vegan or at least to opt for dairy-free milks such as almond, rice and coconut. These milks are now readily available on supermarket shelves as well as in health and wholefood stores. Industry experts say that demand for dairy-free products has doubled in the last five years, highlighting the popularity of reducing or eliminating dairy from the diet. Some 25 million people – nearly half the UK population – have a food intolerance, and dairy is the most common. One school of thought suggests it is because we're overloading our bodies daily with dairy. With cereal and milk as a popular breakfast choice, coffee shop lattes, cheese sandwiches, creamy sauces, yoghurts, milk chocolate and ice cream all common features in the modern diet, it is easy to lose track of the dairy we are regularly consuming. The dairy that we have readily available to us on supermarket shelves are largely processed through the pasteurisation process. This process turns a pure, raw product into an acid-forming food.

Dairy is an acid-forming food. This may come as a surprise; you have possibly heard that drinking a glass of milk can relieve heartburn, when it will actually stimulate the stomach to produce more acid. To optimise health and reduce internal inflammation, acid-forming foods are to be minimised.

I am frequently visited by parents who bring their children for food intolerance testing because they are desperate to find out if any of their conditions are exacerbated by something in their diet. When the conditions in question are asthma, eczema, acne, psoriasis or other skin irritations, I generally advise immediate elimination of dairy for a two-week period prior to the test. This is because dairy can stimulate the production and secretion of mucus, which will aggravate respiratory conditions such as asthma. Also, with the skin being the body's largest detoxification organ, eczema is often one of the first signs of a reaction against dairy foods. In many instances eliminating dairy for 14 days can dramatically reduce symptoms. Sometimes a food intolerance test is still necessary because a dairy-free fortnight does not bring relief from symptoms. With dairy being the number one detected food intolerance, it is a worthwhile suggestion to eliminate without a test, although there is no absolute guarantee that this will be the culprit.

The main concern voiced when I advise clients to reduce or eliminate dairy is calcium deficiency, as they have been led to believe that dairy is needed for strong, healthy bones. First, let me reassure you that there is an abundance of calcium in leafy green vegetables. Secondly, countries with the highest dairy consumption also have the highest rate of osteoporosis. The International Osteoporosis Foundation states that the USA and Europe account for 51% of all fractures from osteoporosis, and they are also the highest and second highest milk consumers in the world. These statistics are no coincidence, as despite what we have been led to believe, pasteurised dairy is contributing to bone damage due to a process known as buffering. When we consume acid-forming foods such as dairy, our body will work hard to restore homeostasis to the pH balance. A high acidity level in the body is called acidosis, and osteoporosis is just one of the chronic conditions linked to it. To counteract acidity, the body will leach alkaline from other places, one of which is the bones. Bones that have consistently been used to buffer pH balance will eventually become weak and lead to osteoporosis.

Furthermore, the use of hormones and antibiotics in the dairy industry will be disrupting endocrines and weakening the immune system and the gut microbiome. Read more about this in the chapter entitled Decrease Your Toxic Load.

My overall advice regarding dairy is to reduce consumption if you are suffering from an inflammatory condition of any kind. In terms of eating clean, your use of dairy will very much depend on where you are on your own rainbow bridge. For most it is easy to switch to a non-dairy milk and only consume occasional natural yoghurt and grass-fed butter. This is where I started on my own clean eating rainbow bridge when I decided for my family and myself to minimise both gluten and dairy.

Although clean eating can be simplified by looking closer at better alternatives to macronutrients, it is not a 'one-size fits all' plan. We each have our own nutrition journeys to embark on, which will start at different places, so progress at your individual pace as you decide how you would like to cross your rainbow bridge.

In order to simultaneously assist multiple clients who have decided to embark on their clean eating journey I virtually mentor a private group twice a year. For 30 days the group eats a diet free from gluten, wheat, dairy and added sugar, using my guidance and support with recipes, menu plans and shopping lists. Although most are initially worried about lack of choice and hunger during the thirty days, the resounding feedback is that they learn an entirely new way of eating and are blown away by the energy and results they access. Most continue to adapt their lifestyle and diet beyond the thirty days. I first ran this group in May 2016 with 140 people in an online support group. At the end of May they had lost a combined weight of 70 stone and were all reporting a significant increase in energy and vitality.

ACTION POINTS

- Choose unprocessed foods, which are close to nature

- Shop mainly in the fruit, vegetable and meat sections of the supermarket

- Swap your macronutrients using the table in this chapter

- Reduce your gluten and dairy intake or eliminate if you are suffering from inflammation

PROPER PREPARATION

'By failing to prepare you are preparing to fail'
BENJAMIN FRANKLIN

This chapter will help if you are:

- A disorganised food shopper

- Shopping for you and your family without any
planning

- Looking for inspiration on what to feed your family
each meal time

If you use social media you may have come across images of an
entire week's worth of meals, arranged in containers with the
slogan 'prepping like a boss' blazoned across them. Prepping like
a boss is the phrase used to describe spending your weekend
planning and preparing your meals and snacks for the week
ahead, to ensure that you avoid temptation and maximise your
health and fitness progression. While this may be a useful concept
for many fitness enthusiasts, it is far from realistic for most
people, especially busy parents who have an entire family to feed.
Even if a busy person with three children and a partner managed

to find enough time and Tupperware to prepare an entire week's meals, is this a sustainable habit that can easily be implemented into everyday life? I'm not so sure. Not to mention the fact that when Wednesday comes around and you don't fancy the dinner you have prepped, you will be reaching for a takeaway menu quicker than you can say 'prepping like a boss'. Furthermore, psychologically we crave what we perceive to be off limits, so this way of eating will surely lead to heightened desire to eat 'off plan'. As a holistic health coach, I also have serious concerns regarding the storage of food in plastic containers. Although Tupperware as a brand have been free from BPA (Bisphenol A) since 2010, most of the cheap plastic storage boxes on the market are not. Plastics such as Bisphenol A (BPA) and Bisphenol S (BPS) have been shown to have hormone-mimicking, estrogenic properties. If you are continually exposed to this material, commonly used in water bottles, canned food and other food containers, you are risking xenoestrogens, which are a danger for oestrogen-fed cancers.

Planning a weekly menu is far too important to do in a rush. I get quite upset when I overhear people saying that they are just 'popping' to the supermarket to 'grab' some shopping. I believe that the time you spend selecting your food shopping is some of the most important of the entire week. It is not something that should be done without planning or taken lightly. The responsibility of a food shop is huge, particularly if you have a family. The food that makes it into your shopping basket will eventually end up in your body, so your choices are either feeding illness or wellness, and there really is no grey area. If it is your responsibility to decide how to fuel your family, give it the time and respect it deserves by preparing. The golden rule regarding preparation is never to attempt food shopping without a list. If written correctly, a shopping list will ensure that you make the best possible choices for you and your family whilst in the supermarket. I advise my clients to begin to create a shopping list by first creating a weekly menu plan, following the 7-7-7 rule when writing their list – seven breakfasts, seven lunches, seven dinners and enough healthy snacks for the next seven days. The ingredients required for the meals in the weekly menu plan will then create your full and final shopping list. There is no need to overthink this process by deciding which days of the week you will consume each meal; the key fact is you have taken time to think about the meals you will eat and have ensured that you have all of the necessary ingredients. This allows you to have freedom of choice on each day and takes the stress out of pre-meal time decision making. It will also eradicate unnecessary and rushed mid-week supermarket trips made because of disorganised dinners and lack of planning. It is on these trips that you are far more likely to buy more than you need and give into the other temptations on offer in the store. On this note, if you find it difficult to complete your food shopping without a few unhealthy additions or you can't resist the smell of the bakery section, I would recommend shopping online instead.

When I explain the 7-7-7 concept to clients they are often concerned about the time this planning might take. I agree that initially this level of organisation can be time-consuming. However, it is well worth investing time in the planning of your family's food choices. Each week, file away your menu plan and shopping list to be recycled and used again. Once you have completed eight consecutive weeks of using the 7-7-7 method you will have two months' worth of menus and corresponding shopping lists on file that can be selected each week without any time taken at all.

When I work with clients on one-to-one basis to assist them in implementing better eating habits, I provide a short recipe book to inspire their choices. I also supply a menu plan and shopping list for the first week as a template to demonstate how best to shop and eat.

In this chapter I have included a few simple recipes as examples of balanced, clean eating meals. I have also included a sample menu plan for one week, as well as the shopping list that corresponds to this plan. On my website (www.mindandbodydetox.co.uk) you can download and print a blank menu template to help you create your weekly meal plans and shopping lists.

When devising your weekly menu, it is beneficial to understand and apply the 80/20 concept. 80/20 is a very simple way to exercise moderation as opposed to deprivation when developing better dietary habits. I live by the 80/20 concept and I encourage my clients to do the same, as it is not only healthy for the body, but also a sound mindset that will provoke a better relationship with food.

The 80/20 concept suggests: 80% of the time you are making the best possible choices for you and your body, while the remaining 20% can be reserved for less healthy options that would be strictly off-limits in most mainstream 'diets'. If you have ever been on a so-called diet, you will be well aware that when a food is restricted and placed off limits you feel completely deprived and begin to crave the exact food you have been told you cannot have. This is one of the many reasons why mainstream diets do not work in the long-term and one of the other major reasons being that most are not designed to work in the long-term. The diet industry is worth £2 billion in the UK alone, the US weight loss market was worth $64 billion in 2014 and 'how to lose weight' is one of the most googled questions. This highly lucrative industry does not want you to succeed in the long-term, and if dieting really worked you'd only need to do it once. The US Federal Trade Commission indicates that diets have a 98% failure rate, which equals repeat custom and huge earnings for the industry that preys on the vulnerable and often desperate.

Living by the 80/20 concept is certainly not a diet that will only last until you have reached your goal. Instead, it is the implementation of healthy habits that will eventually become a lifestyle; a way of enjoying all foods without feelings of depravation, guilt or shame and little chance of weight gain.

When writing your meal plans for the week, take time to ensure that you have chosen at least 80% of healthy foods. The corresponding shopping list should then automatically be at least 80% of healthy ingredients, which will effectively mean that 80% of the foods in your fridge and ultimately your body will be providing you and your family with the necessary fuel you require to optimise your health. When you are certain that you are making healthy choices 80% of the time, you will not feel any guilt or shame when you allow yourself an occasional indulgence, equating to the remaining 20%.

Use these recipes, menu plan and shopping list to inspire your own menus and lists.

BREAKFAST INSPIRATIONS

Mashed avocado and poached egg on toasted rye bread

2 slices of rye bread, toasted
1 avocado, mashed
1 egg, poached

Top with a pinch of good quality sea salt such as Himalayan or Celtic and a crack of black pepper.

Powershake: breakfast on the go

2 handfuls of frozen berries
(strawberries/blueberries/raspberries)
250ml of almond or coconut milk
1 tbsp of coconut flakes
1 handful of raw spinach
1 tsp of coconut oil
2 scoops of vegan protein powder

Blend all ingredients together and enjoy with one palmful of almonds or cashew nuts to eat. This will ensure your metabolism is ignited through the process of chewing.

LUNCH INSPIRATIONS

Grilled turkey and cranberry salad

1 medium turkey breast, grilled
¼ cucumber, sliced
6 cherry tomatoes
2 handfuls of raw spinach
¼ red onion
2 tbsp of cranberries (fresh or dried)
2 tbsp of pine nuts
Dressing: 1 tbsp of olive oil, juice of ½ lemon, black pepper

Butternut squash, quinoa and pecan salad

½ butternut squash, roasted
¼ cup of quinoa, cooked
6 pecan nuts
2 handfuls of rocket leaves
6 cherry tomatoes
½ red onion
Dressing: 1 tbsp of olive oil, juice of 1 lime, black pepper, pinch of Celtic sea salt

DINNER INSPIRATIONS

Chicken, asparagus and cashew nut stir fry

3 tbsp of coconut oil, to cook

2 skinless organic chicken breasts (cut into strips, add to wok and brown)

50g unsalted cashew nuts

4 handfuls of spinach

4 bok choy

2 long red chilies

6 spring onions

250g mange tout

250g asparagus

2 tablespoons of chia seeds

Juice of 1 lime, to dress and garnish

Add coconut oil to wok, add chicken to wok and brown, add all vegetables and cook for 5 minutes, top with chia seeds and lime juice before serving. Tamari sauce is a better alternative to Soy if required.

Sweet potato veggie burger and healthy coleslaw

1 large sweet potato, cooked

170g pinto beans

2 onions, diced

50g rolled oats (preferably gluten-free)

Black pepper and sea salt to taste

2 teaspoons of Worcestershire sauce

Mix ingredients, separate into four patties and cook in oven for 20 minutes on 200c/400f.

Healthy Coleslaw

2 cups of grated cabbage

1 grated carrot

¼ cup of almond mayonnaise (or gluten-free mayonnaise)

1 tbsp apple cider vinegar

1 pinch of Himalayan or Celtic sea salt

Mix all ingredients together before serving with a spoonful of hummus.

SNACKING INSPIRATIONS

If you find yourself hungry between meals, it is okay to snack, as long as you are making good snack choices. However, ensure you are actually hungry and not just thirsty, as many of us do not drink enough water and are confusing thirst for hunger. To calculate whether you are drinking enough water use the calculation: 0.033 x your weight in kg = litres of water to be drunk throughout the day, without taking exercise into consideration. Below is a non-exhaustive list of examples of healthy snack choices.

- Vegetable crudités (carrots/pepper/celery) with 2 tbsp of hummus or guacamole
- 1 piece of fruit and a palmful of nuts (almond/cashew/brazil)
- 2 x oatcakes with nut butter (almond/cashew/hazelnut)
- Homemade energy balls: (1 scoop of vegan protein powder, 1 tbsp of nut butter, flaxseed, cinnamon coconut flakes and 1 tbsp of tahini – simply mix, roll and eat). Mixture makes 6 small balls
- Non-dairy yoghurts with berries – Coyo is a delicious brand

ONE WEEK'S SAMPLE MENU

There is not a 'one size fits all' for diet and nutrition, as we are as unique and individual as our fingerprints. It would be impossible to devise a week's menu to suit each and every reader. However, to give you a better picture of the choices you will be making for improved health, I have created a sample menu for one week. The majority of my clients have busy schedules through work, parenting or both. I believe it is imperative to devise recipes and menus that fit into your week with ease, in order to achieve sustainable results. With this in mind and to save time and money, I am a huge advocate of making big dishes for dinner with a view to having the leftovers for lunch the following day.

PROPER PREPARATION

	Breakfast	Snack	Lunch	Snack	Dinner
Monday	Porridge oats with almond milk, cinnamon, almonds and berries	2 gluten-free oatcakes with almond butter	Grilled fish or chicken, salad and half an avocado	2 tbsp of hummus and raw veg	Stir-fry fish or chicken and plenty of veg, topped with chia and flax seeds
Tuesday	2 poached eggs, spinach, cherry tomatoes and rye bread	Banana and a palmful of almonds	Stir-fry leftovers from Monday	Guacamole with celery	Grilled chicken with added herbs and spices to taste, with brown rice, kale and asparagus
Wednesday	Grainless granola with Coyo yoghurt and berries	Vegan protein shake	Vegetable omelette with a small green side salad and pine nuts	2 oatcakes with nut butter	Homemade burgers, sweet potato wedges topped with turmeric and homemade coleslaw
Thursday	Mashed avocado on rye bread topped with a poached egg	Sliced apple dipped in 1 tbsp of almond butter	Tuna Nicoise salad topped with sunflower seeds	Palmful of cashew nuts and 1 piece of fruit	Sticky salmon or chicken (cooked in honey and sesame marinade) roasted veg and brown rice
Friday	Superfood Smoothie and a palmful of nuts	2 tbsp of hummus and raw veg	Thursdays leftover salmon served with a leafy salad	3 homemade energy balls	Courgette Bolognese served with spiralised courgette instead of spaghetti pasta
Saturday	Protein pancakes (1 egg, 1 scoop of protein and almond milk) served with berries	Guacamole and celery sticks	Friday's leftover courgette bolognese	Coyo yoghurt with cinnamon and berries	White fish served with steamed veg and quinoa
Sunday	Porridge with almond milk, berries, cinnamon and crushed almonds	1 vegan protein shake	Homemade tomato soup with a leafy green side salad and pine nuts	2 oatcakes with almond butter	Traditional Sunday roast, with roast potatoes cooked in coconut oil (avoid Yorkshire pudding)

To make salads and vegetables more interesting: try adding extra virgin olive oil, pumpkin seed oil, or sesame seed oil, or make your own dressing by adding wholegrain mustard, apple cider vinegar, balsamic vinegar or lemon juice and fresh or dried herbs with sea salt and black pepper

SHOPPING LIST

Some suggestions for a more nutritious shopping list:

- Choose organic when possible, especially grains, meat, dairy and root vegetables. Remember, food that is the most fragile or has to look the most presentable, e.g. strawberries, lettuce, will be the most heavily sprayed. (See the clean fifteen and dirty dozen list in the Decrease Your Toxic Load chapter)
- Choose foods in season where possible and include a variety of colours. Use raw vegetables where possible as they are rich in enzymes that can aid digestion

STORE CUPBOARD STAPLES

Regardless of what appears on your shopping list each week, I highly recommend that you maintain stock of the following items to ensure that you always have healthy choices on hand to accompany and flavour dishes.

Grains: brown basmati rice, buckwheat, millet, quinoa

Nuts: almonds, brazils, cashews, hazelnuts, pecans, pine nuts and walnuts

Seeds: flax, pumpkin, sesame and sunflower

Breads and crackers: rye bread, Nairn's gluten-free oatcakes

Seasonings: fresh and dried herbs, sea salt, pepper, Braggs' liquid aminos (soya sauce alternative), apple cider vinegar, lemon, lime, chilli, ginger, spices, onion salt and garlic salt, cinnamon, nutmeg, mixed herbs

Oils: extra virgin olive oil, (*not to cook with, but add to food after cooking or as a dressing*), coconut oil

Cupboard basics: lentils, chickpeas, butterbeans, cartons of tomatoes

Freezer basics: mixed berries, raspberries, blueberries, pineapple

Fridge basics: fresh vegetables, almond or cashew nut butters, organic free-range eggs

SAMPLE MENU – SHOPPING LIST

Fruit and vegetables

Spinach, rocket, avocados, cucumber, tomatoes, beetroot, peppers, onions, beansprouts, courgettes, mushrooms, carrots, kale, asparagus, celery, sweet potatoes, potatoes, bananas, green beans, blueberries, broccoli, strawberries, garlic, mange tout, apples, cabbage, lemons, mango, chilli, raspberries

Meat

Chicken breasts, whole chicken, salmon fillet, turkey mince, cod fillet, king prawns, beef mince

Fridge

Almond butter, almond milk, hummus, guacamole, eggs, cashew butter, Coyo yoghurts

Spice Rack

Turmeric, cinnamon, garlic salt, rosemary, mixed herbs, Celtic sea salt, black pepper

Cupboard

Nairn's gluten-free oatcakes, coconut oil, quinoa, extra virgin olive oil, apple cider vinegar, coconut flakes, cartons of tomatoes, brown rice, rye bread, gluten free mayo, granola, olives, tuna in spring water

Nuts and seeds

Cashews, brazils, pine nuts, hazelnuts, pecans, almonds, sunflower seeds, pumpkin seeds, chia seeds, milled flax seeds

Becoming disciplined about shopping and no longer disorganised about your food choices will provide a multitude of benefits. Although you will initially need to invest time in adopting the 7-7-7 method for a menu plan and shopping list, this process will ultimately save you time. Not only can weekly lists be recycled, but also once you have built an 8-week collection the list will enable you to select your items quickly without wasting time looking for goods that you do not need, as an uninspired shopper so often does.

Believe it or not, proper preparation regarding your weekly

menu will actually mean less stress in the long run. As this discipline becomes a habit (which won't take long) you will no longer be left to figure out what to cook and whether you have the correct ingredients. Just follow the list and relax in the knowledge that you have adopted a stress-free and well-organised approach to food prep.

Research suggests that a shopping list can reduce your food expenses by up to 25% if you do not deviate from it. Supermarkets are designed to make you spend your hard-earned money, with the most profitable products placed at eye level, and the store layout ensures the most frequently purchased items are separated around the store, making you walk the entire distance and tempting you to make additional purchases. Having a well-thought out list that you trust has all you need will ensure you do not fall victim to the marketing tricks of these stores.

The biggest benefit to preparing a weekly food menu and shopping list is the opportunity it provides to evaluate how healthy your diet is. It is far easier to apply the 80/20 concept of clean eating when you have listed what you will be consuming and can make necessary amendments before it is even purchased. It is also the perfect opportunity to gather input from family members and is one of the tools I use to educate my children on making better choices.

ACTION POINTS

- Visit www.mindandbodydetox.co.uk to download blank weekly menu templates

- Complete a blank weekly menu template using the recipes in this section for inspiration and the 7-7-7 method

- Using your weekly menu, compile a shopping list of everything you need for the week

- Ensure you have applied the 80/20 concept to your weekly list, making any necessary amendments

QUICK BURSTS - HIIT SESSIONS AT HOME

This chapter has been written by Mind and Body Detox Co-Founder,
personal trainer and health coach, James Dunne.

'Movement is a medicine for creating change in a
person's physical, emotional and mental states'
CAROL WELCH

This chapter will help if you:

- Want to be able to work out in the comfort of your
  own home

- Can only spare 20 minutes a day to exercise

- Want to burn fat, become leaner and increase
  muscle definition

Movement is a key ingredient in wellbeing, which is why I
encourage clients to move more. This doesn't mean daily visits
to the gym for excessive workouts. In fact, in some instances we
would simply recommend walking to increase daily movement,
particularly if a client hadn't exercised at all for several years.
Most people in today's world spend far too much time sitting due
to desk work and 'down' time in front of the TV or computer.

If you are one of those people who sit at a desk for eight hours a day, only moving to visit the bathroom, you are in good company.

I encourage clients to increase their daily non-exercise activity thermogenesis (NEAT). This is the energy expended on everything we do that isn't sleeping or a sports-like exercise. I have a reminder on my phone to get up and walk around for a little, every 45 minutes. This helps to create clarity of what I am doing and increases my daily NEAT. Any physical activity completed will increase your metabolic rate substantially. The cumulative impact over a week, month and beyond can have a significant positive outcome on the body's ability to burn more calories and store less fat.

Several clients have come to me with endocrine disorders. The endocrine system influences how your heart beats and how bones and tissues grow. It can play an integral role in whether or not you develop diabetes, thyroid disease, growth disorders and a host of other hormone conditions. Many people believe that they have a 'slow metabolism'. This may be due to the cumulative effect of many years' lack of movement and non-stop yo-yo dieting.

Many people think that as long as they go to the gym several times a week this will suffice. I agree that this can be an ideal way to expend calories, however, there are several ways to burn them throughout the day without strenuous exercise. Weight management can be made easier with the understanding of NEAT.

Below are some effective means to burn additional calories each day.

- Playing with the children
- Walking the dog

- Chores in the garden
- Washing the car
- Food shopping
- Getting off the bus or train a stop earlier and walking
- Walking upstairs to use the bathroom

If you are a fan of self-development talks, plug in an audio and take a power walk.

If you are at home on the phone, walk around completing other tasks whilst on the phone (wearing headphones, rather than holding the phone, lowering phone radiation exposure to the brain).

If you are sitting at a desk for most of the day, try to conduct meetings outside rather than in a meeting room or boardroom, as you also tend to be more creative this way. If the weather is sunny, you will also be increasing your vitamin D, the sunshine vitamin.

Research suggest that individuals who move constantly throughout the day are more likely to reach their desired weight goals than people who have a sedentary job and vigorously move through exercise in one main session.

Researcher James Levine, MD, who published many journal reports on the effects on NEAT found that adopting such methods can increase your daily calorie expenditure by as much as 350 calories per day, and is most beneficial for obese individuals.

NEAT is the proof that the compound effect works. As covered throughout the book, simple healthy habits and daily disciplines over time can make a dramatic difference to your health and, as a by-product, to your waistline too. Try and incorporate some of the above into your daily routine.

If you have already mastered this and want to move on to the next level, then HIIT training is a great starting point.

HIIT (High Intensity Interval Training) has become very popular in recent times and it is easy to see why. This method of training will help improve bone density, strength, lean muscle mass and the release of endorphins will have a positive effect on your overall mood, boosted metabolism, effective fat burning modality, improved insulin resistance and improvements in cardiovascular health.

It is a great source of exercise for pretty much anyone, anywhere. The parent at home for most of the day, the business person living out of hotels or the person who wants to train whilst on holiday.

HIIT typically involves short bursts of very intensive exercise followed by short recovery phases, i.e. 40 seconds of hard work and 20 seconds of rest. This type of workout is extremely effective for fat burning and fat loss, especially if you add further resistance training in the form of weights. I prefer to offer this modality to clients compared to the 'steady state cardio'.

We are made up of trillions of cells and all have our own unique DNA.' 'DNA Fit' is a test that I offer my clients, as it helps eliminate the guesswork, since DNA consists of the building blocks of the body. It is your genetic blueprint to navigate you towards the right decisions for your goals. The test is suitable for beginners, advanced athletes or people that want to live healthier lives. Whether you're looking to increase muscle, decrease body fat or want to optimise your nutrition, your genetics hold valuable information about the best way to do this. Each individual responds to exercise, recovery and food in different ways, and having an understanding of this will give you a tremendous indication of long-term, sustainable results. For more information on the DNA Fit Test, visit my website: http://www.mindandbodydetox.co.uk/index/readblog/34

I believe that most forms of training have their place and it is advisable to try as many as possible for a period of time to see which one appears to get the best results and which is the one that you most enjoy. If you are not motivated and not enjoying your fitness training, the less likely you are to do it.

Steady cardio for prolonged periods of time can promote muscle loss and can be catabolic (muscle tissue and essential fat deposits found within the body can become depleted). Due to the constant pounding of the road or treadmills, prolonged steady cardio can cause you to age faster, affect joints and cause hormones to be out of balance. Hours spent on the treadmill can decrease testosterone and raise levels of the stress hormone, cortisol. Increased levels of cortisol can stimulate appetite and potentially increase fat storage. If cardio is your preferred method of training then ensure that you vary the speed, incline, time, etc.

'Steady state cardio' will enable you to burn a high amount of calories whilst exercising, but as soon as you stop, your calorie burning stops too. In contrast, HIIT will burn calories whilst exercising and up to 36-48 hours after exercise, creating a unique metabolic response in your body.

This is known as exercise post oxygen consumption (EPOC), or the 'afterburn' affect. The analogy between steady state cardio and bodyweight/resistance/strength training is that, in my experience, most people would prefer to have the appearance of a 100m runner than a marathon runner. Therefore, it is best to train as a 100m would, through short, sharp intense sprints and explosive work, rather than prolonged steady state running. If you desire to have a lean, strong, athletic appearance then resistance training is advisable. Muscle cells are up to eight times more metabolically active than fat cells. Therefore, the more muscle you have, the more calories you will burn at both rest and during exercise.

One element of training that I recommend to clients is to incorporate hill-sprint interval training, post-strength work a couple of times a week. Many more fatty acids will be released into the bloodstream for energy after resistance training. When free fatty acids are released from the fat cell, it shrinks and that's why you look leaner. When you lose body fat, the fat cell has reduced.

HIIT PREPARATION

To prevent injury when exercising make sure that you carry out some initial warming up and stretching as well as a cool-down once you have finished. Also ensure that you have plenty of water on standby. Ideally use a BPA-free bottle of water, and in order to continually keep the body hydrated, only drink water at room temperature and not ice-cold water. As Paul Chek suggests in his book *How to eat, move and be healthy*, try this interesting experiment. Drink a large glass of cold water, jump up and down and you will feel the water sloshing around your stomach. Whereas if you drink a glass at room temperature it will be immediately assimilated into your body without the sloshing sound.

HERE COMES THE HIIT

No gym membership is necessary, as these exercises can be completed in the comfort of your own home without any equipment.

The exercise description with 'regression' allows for modifications if the initial exercises are too challenging to begin with. Put on some music and get to work. Do the ten exercises below and repeat.

A warm-up is often overlooked, but jumping straight into high-level activity can be detrimental. Warming up stimulates blood flow and releases synovial fluid, which helps to lubricate the joints and increases your mental readiness for the workout.

With this kind of workout, a suitable warm-up would be some dynamic stretching in the form of marching on the spot, arm circles, leg swings, squats and lunges for 3-5 minutes.

Beginners – work for 20 seconds with 40 seconds rest

Intermediates – work for 30 seconds and 30 seconds rest

Advanced – work for 40 seconds with 20 seconds rest

With every exercise, engage your core (the muscles in your torso) and really think about what muscles you are working, also known as the mind muscle connection (MMC). It is often easy to just go through the motions of an exercise. By focusing on the muscles you are working, you can recruit a greater number of muscle fibres. Focus on each rep in the targeted muscle group.

1. Running on the spot (high knees)

Shoulders relaxed, land and take off on toes, engage with arms.

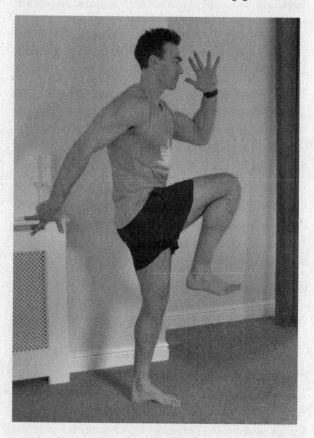

Regression – one step at a time, walking effect.

2. Press-ups

On tiptoes, elbows soft, back straight, weight over hands, core tight.

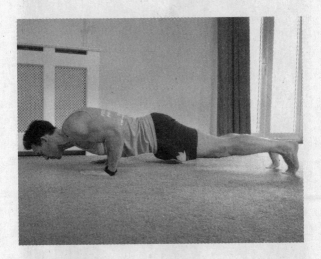

Regression – knees on floor.

3. Jumping squats

Back straight, weights on heels, engage core.

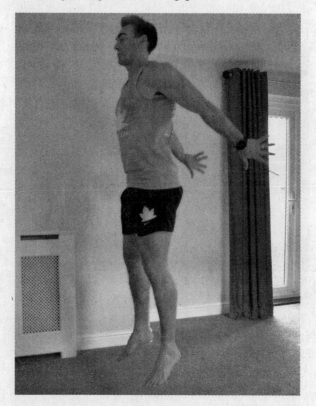

Explode upwards and land softly on toes.

Regression (air squats), feet remain on the floor throughout.

4. Tricep dips with legs extended

Body remains still, only bend arms, keep bottom up, tight core.

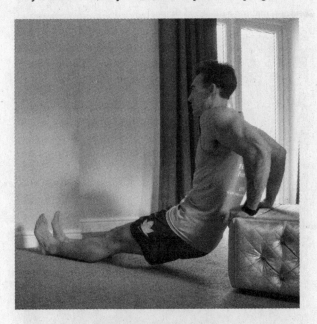

Regression – legs much closer to the torso and/or in a box shape with heels flat on the floor.

5. Diamond jacks

Explode upwards, heels to touch inside each other, land lightly on toes, making a diamond shape.

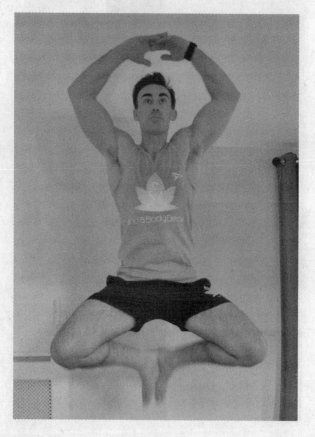

Regression – star jumps, with a much smaller jump.

6. Jumping lunges

Feet staggered, propel one leg forward, switching the position of your feet mid-air, landing softly.

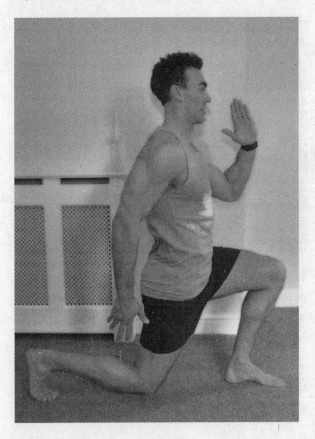

Regression – lunges without a jump.

7. Chest to floor and get up

From a standing position, jump backwards and land into a low press-up position.

Jump up and forward to land in squat position, stand up and re-set.

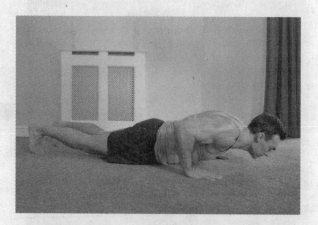

Regression – from kneeling, step out one foot at a time, rather than jump. The same applies when coming back up to stand, one foot at a time.

8. Uppercut punch with engaging twist

Exaggerate the twist working the obliques, (located either side of the abdomen) clench your fist as tight as possible, creating greater tension in the arms.

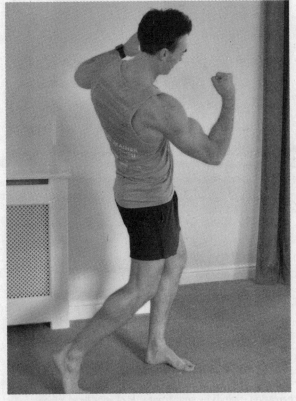

Regression – uppercut without the twist.

9. Tuck jumps

Legs slightly narrower than shoulder width apart, explode upwards and bring knees into chest, land as softly as possible.

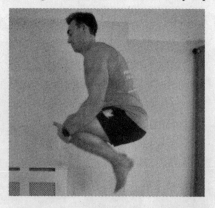

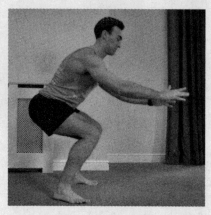

Regression – hands by your front side of your head, elbows flaring out and one knee at a time to hit same side of elbow.

10. Donkey kick

Begin in a high plank position, engage core, flick both legs up and touch bottom, land lightly on toes and repeat.

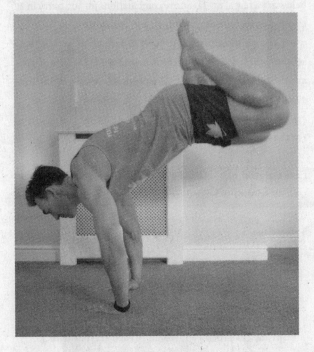

Regression – one leg up at a time and repeat.

If you are a beginner, within a short number of HIIT sessions, you will soon be able to increase both the time of work and the intensity.

Below are a few of my favourite combinations for you to try in 20 minutes or so, excluding warm up and cool down.

If you are a beginner, start with 20 seconds of work with 40 seconds of rest and then you can slowly increase the time of work and decrease the time of rest: 30 seconds on, 30 seconds off; then 40 seconds on and 20 seconds off.

For the more advanced, try some of these combinations.

Here's a good one – called Tabata it's when you alternate 20 seconds on with 10 seconds rest.

5 exercises

- 1st set 10 secs of each exercise x 5 is 50 seconds' work, 10 seconds' rest
- 2nd set 20 secs of each exercise, 20 seconds' rest and so on. Up to 50 seconds per exercise
- 3rd and final round 30 seconds of each exercise with 30 seconds' rest

Another progression is a HIIT pyramid: 2 x squats, 2 x sit ups, 2 x squat jumps, 3 x squats, 3 x sit ups, 3 x jump squats and so on up to 15. If you have time, work all the way back down to one.

If you are really gaining strength and energy, try this one: 5

exercises 90 seconds each, 30 secs rest in between and repeat. Choose from the below list of exercises and mix it up each time so that you are working different muscle groups in each HIIT session.

- Clap press ups
- Semi-circle mountain climbers
- Chest to floor get up and tuck jump
- Squat thrusts
- Low skater jumps
- Archer press ups
- One arm burpees
- Jumping lunges on each leg and jump squat
- Blast press-up
- High donkey kick

Once completed, make sure that you de-stretch with a cool down. I always encourage clients to do this sitting down, as it helps regulate the heart rate slightly faster and will reduce delayed onset muscle soreness (DOMS). Stretching will help to release tension from the workout. Hold each stretch for 20–30 seconds for each of the major muscle groups – quads, hamstrings, calves, shoulders, back, chest.

HIIT doesn't simply mean bodyweight exercises. There are a variety of other modalities that we can implement this for too. Try as many options as you can and see which one you enjoy the most.

- Treadmill HIIT
- Boxing
- Plyometric jumps

- Kettlebells
- Dumbbells

Low-intensity steady state (LISS) is a great modality if you are new to HIIT training, as the exercise is unlikely to impede recovery when your muscles are sore. Examples of LISS are walking, swimming and cycling at a relaxed, lower intensity. This type of exercise can help to increase blood flow to damaged cells and reduce DOMS. Furthermore, it doesn't add additional stress to the body if completed several times a week (above four hours throughout the week). This type of exercise can burn very little muscle and a lot of fat.

With exercise, getting started is the hardest part, and the thought is often far worse than the process. However, once you begin to feel the benefits of boosted energy levels, raised endorphins, elevated moods and loss of body fat you will find it easy to implement this as a healthy habit. Just 20 minutes of HIIT training, three times a week can, and will make a big difference to your health and shape. Be consistent, be motivated, be proud and above all else enjoy it.

ACTION POINTS

- If you are new to exercise, begin with the NEAT and simply move more

- Twice a week get up 30 minutes earlier than you usually do to allow for a warm up, a HIIT session and cool-down to start the day on a positive step

- Once you begin to build strength and stamina, challenge yourself with the progression exercises in this chapter

- Take regular long walks and enjoy the fresh air

MIRACLE

Take action, have faith, create miracles

I have shared my own journey of finding strength in adversity. The death of my parents had a profound effect on me, that's for sure. I could have allowed the experience to harden me and the pain to make me resentful, but I wasn't prepared to allow bitterness to steal my sweetness. Overcoming life's obstacles is never easy – it takes grit, determination and faith that darkness will eventually lead into light. To climb my mountain I used the tools I have given you throughout this book to strengthen both my mind and body. By taking action, and by having complete faith in the outcome I have learnt that at the top of every mountain is a miracle.

Hal Elrod, author of *The Miracle Morning*, says:

'The moment you take responsibility for everything in your life is the moment you can change anything in your life.'

I could have read this quote and questioned how on earth I could take responsibility for the death of my mum and dad just five days apart. Of course, I cannot take responsibility for their passing, but I can take responsibility for how it impacts on me and my own happiness. Initially I was angry and felt cheated that I had lost my parents possibly 20 years too soon – who wouldn't be? However, remembering my mum telling me that I couldn't spend the rest of my life feeling hurt and resentful when she had gone, meant I had to take action. Finding and implementing daily disciplines to cultivate a healthier mindset gave me the self-belief, motivation and faith I needed in my darkest hours. I gained clarity through meditation and became grateful for all that I had, instead of dwelling on all that I had lost. I learned to let go of the things I couldn't change and focus on the things I could and would change.

Putting into practice the healthy habits I was learning through my nutrition training gave me the ability to heal my body, a strong vehicle to carry me up that mountain. I healed my autoimmune condition by restoring my gut health and I became completely aware of what I was exposing my body to. I fuelled my body with the correct nutrition it was craving then instilled these values into my family so that we could all experience the benefits of clean eating.

I wanted to share my toolkit because I know that life isn't plain sailing, and when those waters get choppy we need to know how to navigate them. I don't have super powers, and I'm not an exception to the rules of adversity – I simply had faith that I could get through the worst and took action to do so – and you can too.

This book was designed so you do not need to read it in order, or all at once. This was important because I know in overwhelming times we do not also need to be overwhelmed with information. By reading the chapters that resonate the most with you and implementing the action points, you are already beginning to create your own miracle. Although you may feel that the action you are taking is small and insignificant, have faith that applied consistently over time you will see the results. Also give yourself credit for executing the action points and having faith in the process, as I know some will read this book and expect miracles from that alone.

No-one is coming to save us, but that's fine because why should we task anyone else with that much responsibility? Especially when we have all we need to save ourselves. Don't wait for a miracle – be one. You have everything you need now. Inside your mind and inside your body, there lies a miracle.

Take action, have faith and go and create miracles. The world is waiting for the best *you*.

REFERENCES

DAILY AFFIRMATIONS

Emotional vitality and incident coronary heart disease: benefits of healthy psychological functioning, 2007 by LD Kubzansky and RC Thurston, Harvard School of Public Health:
https://www.ncbi.nlm.nih.gov/pubmed/18056547

ATTITUDE OF GRATITUDE

Robert A Emmons, studies on gratitude:
http://emmons.faculty.ucdavis.edu/gratitude-and-well-being/

Indiana University, The effects of gratitude expression on neural activity by Dr Joshua Brown et al, December 2015:
https://www.indiana.edu/~irf/home/in-the-news/

University of Kentucky, A grateful heart is a non-violent heart by Nathan Dewall et al, 2012: https://goo.gl/xwbHVV

Subjective Well-Being and Adaptation to Life Events: A Meta-Analysis on Differences Between Cognitive and Affective Well-Being by Maike Luhmann et al:
https://www.ncbi.nlm.nih.gov/pmc/articles/PMC3289759/

2011 Applied Psychology Health & Wellbeing, Gratitude & Sleep: www.psychologytoday.com/blog/minding-the-body/201111/how-gratitude-helps-you-sleep-night

MEDITATIONS AND VISUALISATIONS

Meditation for the reduction of anxiety and depression by John Hopkins et al, published in JAMA 2014:
http://www.hopkinsmedicine.org/news/media/releases/meditation_for_anxiety_and_depression

The Journal of Alternative and Complementary Medicine, Meditation and Substance Abuse by Alberto Chiesa. January 2010 16 (1), 37-46: https://doi.org/10.1089/acm.2009.0362

Effects of mindfulness based cognitive therapy on neurophysiological correlates of performance monitoring in adult attention deficit/hyperactivity disorder: www.clinph-journal.com/article/S1388-2457(13)01228-5/abstract?cc=y

Effects of Visualisation on performance of basketball players, March 2013 by Alan Richardson:
http://www.tandfonline.com/doi/abs/10.1080/10671188.1967.10614808

THE POWER OF THE SUBCONSCIOUS MIND

University of Illinois and Texas review on positivity, life
expectancy and improved health: Happy People Live Longer:
Subjective Well-Being

Contributes to Health and Longevity by Ed Diener and Micaela
Chan, October 2010: http://bit.ly/2ubvh77

LET IT GO

Modelling cognition in emotional disorder: the S-REF model
1996 by Adrian Wells of the University of Manchester and
Gerald Matthews of the University of
https://www.ncbi.nlm.nih.gov/pubmed/8990539

YOUR VIBE, YOUR TRIBE

Physical Nature of Vibrations by Dr Bernard Beitman,
University of Missouri:
http://www.theepochtimes.com/n3/668208-is-there-a-
physical-explanation-for-the-vibes-you-get-off-people/

Dr Emoto Masaru vibrational rice experiment:
https://youtu.be/Ehlw-9PJKlE

FIGHT THE FIRE OF INFLAMMATION

The correlation between C-reactive protein and cardiovascular events, Ridker, P M et al published in The New England Journal of Medicine, November 2002. 347(20), 1557-1565: www.nejm.org/doi/full/10.1056/NEJM09021993#t=article

Diet induced metabolic acidosis by Maria M Adeva, Gema Souto published in Clinical Nutrition Journal August 2011 v30, Iss4, pgs 416-421: www.clinicalnutritionjournal.com/article/S0261-5614(11)00060-4/fulltext

Montmorency cherry juice reducing effects of gout by Glyn Howatson, Northumbria University 2014: https://www.northumbria.ac.uk/about-us/news-events/news/2014/09/drinking-montmorency-cherry-concentrate-reduces-effects-of-gout/

Cereal Grains: Humanity's Double-Edged Sword by Dr Loren Cordain, US Colorado State University: www.ncbi.nlm.nih.gov/pubmed/10489816

HEAL YOUR GUT

Common Gut Imbalances in Autistic People by Rosa Krajmalnik-Brown, professor James Adams, US Arizone State University, August 2014: https://asunow.edu/content/asu-experts-follow-gut-reaction-autism-tratment-study

FULL LIST OF CONDITIONS CLASSIFIED AS AUTOIMMUNE

HEART

Myocarditis

Postmyocardial infarction syndrome

Postpericardiotomy syndrome

Subacute bacterial endocarditis (SBE)

Anti-Glomerular Basement Membrane nephritis

Interstitial cystitis

Lupus nephritis

LIVER

Autoimmune hepatitis

Primary biliary cirrhosis(PBC)

Primary sclerosing cholangitis

LUNG

Antisynthetase syndrome

SKIN

Alopecia Areata

Autoimmune Angioedema

Autoimmune progesterone dermatitis

Autoimmune urticaria

Bullous pemphigoid

Cicatricial pemphigoid

Dermatitis herpetiformis

Discoid lupus erythematosus

Epidermolysis bullosa acquisita

Erythema nodosum

Gestational pemphigoid

Hidradenitis suppurativa

Lichen planus

Lichen sclerosus

Linear IgA disease(LAD)

Morphea

Pemphigus vulgaris

Pityriasis lichenoides et varioliformis acuta

Mucha-Habermann disease

Psoriasis

Systemic scleroderma

Vitiligo

ADRENAL GLANDS

Addison's disease

MULTI-GLANDULAR

Autoimmune polyendocrine syndrome (APS) type 1

Autoimmune polyendocrine syndrome (APS) type 2

Autoimmune polyendocrine syndrome (APS) type 3

PANCREAS

Autoimmune pancreatitis(AIP)

Diabetes mellitus type 1

THYROID

Autoimmune thyroiditis

Ord's thyroiditis

Graves' disease

REPRODUCTIVE ORGANS

Autoimmune Oophoritis

Endometriosis

Autoimmune orchitis

SALIVARY GLANDS

Sjogren's syndrome

DIGESTIVE SYSTEM

Autoimmune enteropathy

Coeliac disease

Crohn's disease

Microscopic colitis

Ulcerative colitis

BLOOD

Antiphospholipid syndrome(APS, APLS)

Aplastic anemia

Autoimmune hemolytic anemia

Autoimmune lymphoproliferative syndrome

Autoimmune neutropenia

Autoimmune thrombocytopenic purpura

Cold agglutinin disease

Essential mixed cryoglobulinemia

Evans syndrome

Paroxysmal nocturnal hemoglobinuria

Pernicious anemia

Pure red cell aplasia

Thrombocytopenia

CONNECTIVE TISSUE, SYSTEMIC & MULTIPLE ORGAN

Adiposis dolorosa

Adult-onset Still's disease

Ankylosing Spondylitis

CREST syndrome

Drug-induced lupus

Enthesitis-related arthritis

Eosinophilic fasciitis

Felty syndrome

IgG4-related disease

Juvenile Arthritis

Lyme disease (Chronic)

Mixed connective tissue disease (MCTD)

Palindromic rheumatism

Parry Romberg syndrome

Parsonage-Turner syndrome

Psoriatic arthritis

Reactive arthritis

Relapsing polychondritis

Retroperitoneal fibrosis

Rheumatic fever

Rheumatoid arthritis

Sarcoidosis

Schnitzler syndrome

Systemic Lupus Erythematosus(SLE)

Undifferentiated connective tissue disease (UCTD)

MUSCLE

Dermatomyositis

Fibromyalgia

Inclusion body myositis

Myositis

Myasthenia gravis

Neuromyotonia

Paraneoplastic cerebellar degeneration

Polymyositis

NERVOUS SYSTEM

Acute disseminated encephalomyelitis (ADEM)

Acute motor axonal neuropathy

Anti-N-Methyl-D-Aspartate (Anti-NMDA) Receptor Encephalitis

Balo concentric sclerosis

Bickerstaff's encephalitis

Chronic inflammatory demyelinating polyneuropathy

Guillain–Barré syndrome

Hashimoto's encephalopathy

Idiopathic inflammatory demyelinating diseases

Lambert-Eaton myasthenic syndrome

Multiple sclerosis, pattern II

Oshtoran Syndrome

Paediatric Autoimmune Neuropsychiatric Disorder Associated with Streptococcus (PANDAS)

Progressive inflammatory neuropathy

Restless leg syndrome

Stiff person syndrome

Sydenham chorea

Transverse myelitisEYES

Autoimmune retinopathy

Autoimmune uveitis

Cogan syndrome

Graves ophthalmopathy

Intermediate uveitis

Ligneous conjunctivitis

Mooren's ulcer

Neuromyelitis optica

Opsoclonus myoclonus syndrome

Optic neuritis

Scleritis

Susac's syndrome

Sympathetic ophthalmia

Tolosa-Hunt syndrome

EARS

Autoimmune inner ear disease (AIED)

VASCULAR SYSTEM

Ménière's disease

Behçet's disease

REFERENCES

Eosinophilic granulomatosis with polyangiitis (EGPA)
Giant cell arteritis
Granulomatosis with polyangiitis (GPA)
IgA vasculitis (IgAV)
Kawasaki's disease
Leukocytoclastic vasculitis
Lupus vasculitis
Rheumatoid vasculitis
Microscopic polyangiitis(MPA)
Polyarteritis nodosa (PAN)
Polymyalgia rheumatica
Urticarial vasculitis
Vasculitis

SYSTEMIC
Chronic fatigue syndrome
Complex regional pain syndrome
Eosinophilic esophagitis
Gastritis
Interstitial lung disease
POEMS syndrome
Raynaud's phenomenon
Primary immunodeficiency
Pyoderma gangrenosum

209

FULL LIST OF SYMPTOMS OF A FOOD INTOLERANCE

- Abdominal pains
- Joint pains
- Acid reflux
- Bloating
- Constipation
- Diarrhoea
- IBS
- Nausea
- Stomach cramps
- Arthritis
- Ganglions
- Chronic fatigue syndrome
- Eczema
- Dermatitis
- Rashes
- Urticaria/Hives
- Headaches
- Migraines
- Tension
- Sinusitis
- Constant stuffy nose

- Rhinitis
- Wheezing
- Constant dry cough
- Brain Fog
- Blurred vision
- Flu like body pain
- Itchy Ears or nose
- Unexplained weight gain
- Difficulty losing weight
- Depression
- Mood swings
- Irritability
- Aggressiveness
- Slow growth in children
- Bedwetting in children
- Night terrors in children
- Insomnia
- Anxiety
- Panic Attacks
- PMS
- Tendency to feel cold

Bone Broth Recipe

Ingredients

2 pounds (or more) of bones from organic meat

2 chicken feet for extra gelatin (optional)

1 onion

2 carrots

2 stalks of celery

2 tablespoons Apple Cider Vinegar

Optional: 1 bunch of parsley, 1 tablespoon or more of sea salt, 1 teaspoon peppercorns, additional herbs or spices to taste. I also add 2 cloves of garlic for the last 30 minutes of cooking.

You'll also need a large stock pot or slow cooker to cook the broth in and a strainer to remove the pieces when it is done.

Instructions

1. If you are using raw bones, especially beef bones, it improves the flavour to roast them in the oven first. I place them in a roasting pan and roast for 30 minutes at 350.
2. Then, place the bones in a large stock pot. Pour filtered water over the bones and add the vinegar. Let sit for 20-30 minutes in the cool water. The acid helps make the nutrients in the bones more available.
3. Rough chop and add the vegetables (except the parsley and garlic, if using) to the pot. Add any salt, pepper, spices, or herbs, if using.

4. Now, bring the broth to a boil. Once it has reached a vigorous boil, reduce to a simmer and simmer for the remainder of the 24hr cooking time.

5. During the first few hours of simmering, you'll need to remove the impurities that float to the surface. A frothy/foamy layer will form and it can be easily scooped off with a big spoon. Throw this part away. Check it every 20 minutes for the first 2 hours to remove this.

6. During the last 30 minutes, add the garlic and parsley, if using.

7. Remove from heat and let cool slightly. Strain using a fine metal strainer to remove all the bits of bone and vegetable. When cool enough, store in a gallon size glass jar in the fridge for up to 5 days, or freeze for later use.

FULL LIST OF BENEFICIAL BACTERIA STRAINS AND USES

Lactobacillus Species

The predominant and most important bacteria that reside in the small intestine are the Lactobacillus species.

Strain Name	What It Supports
L. acidophilus	Overall digestion Nutrient absorption Relief from occasional cramping, gas, and diarrhea Immune health Urinary and vaginal health in women
L. fermentum	Overall digestion Detoxification
L. plantarum	Overall digestion Immune health
L. rhamnosus	Traveler's diarrhea Vaginal health in women
L. salivarius	Immune health Oral health
L. paracasei	Liver health
L. gasseri	Vaginal health Relief from occasional diarrhea
L. reuteri	Oral health Immune health Overall digestion

Bifidobacterium Species

Billions of Bifidobacterium line the walls of the large intestine (colon) and help ward off invasive harmful bacteria and other microorganisms, including yeast.

Strain Name	What It Supports
B. bifidum	Overall digestion Nutrient absorption Relief from occasional diarrhea (particularly related to travel)
B. longum	Overall digestion Detoxification Immune health
B. infantis	Overall digestion Relief from occasional bloating and constipation

Bacillus Species

Bacillus bacteria are rod-shaped, spore-bearing bacteria that produce lactic acid. It also resides in the body longer than other bacteria and is excreted slowly.

Strain Name	What It Supports
B. Coagulan	Overall digestion Relief from occasional constipation Vaginal health

Streptoccocus Species

This probiotic strain is found in the oral cavity's mucus membranes and is known for its ability to produce BLIS (bacteriocin-like inhibitory substances),

Strain Name	What It Supports
S. salivarius K12	Overall oral health Immune health Reoccurring throat infections
S. Salivarius M18	Healthy teeth and gums

DECREASE YOUR TOXIC LOAD

Cancerous Levels of Toxins, US University of California:
https://www.ucdmc.ucdavis.edu/publish/news/newsroom/7190

Contribution of Extrinsic Risk Factors to Cancer Development, December 2016 led by Yusuf Hannun, MD, & Joel Strum Kenny at US Stony Brook University New York:
http://sb.cc.stonybrook.edu/news/general/2015-12-16-study-reveals-environment-behavior-contribute-to-some-80-percent-of-cancer.php

The Safety Assessment of Sodium Lauryl Sulfate and Ammonium Lauryl Sulfate published by The Journal of The American College of Toxicology:
journals.sagepub.com/doi/pdf/10.3109/10915818309142005

DIY CLEANING PRODUCTS RECIPES

Toilet Cleaner/Mildew Remover: pour ½ cup of baking soda and 10 drops of tea tree essential oil into the toilet. Add ¼ cup of vinegar to the bowl and scrub while the mixture fizzes.

Bathroom Surface Cleaner: Fill a small spray bottle with 1 cup of white and a few drops of an essential oil of your choosing (lemon and tea tree are my favourite).

All-purpose Cleaner: Mix together equal parts vinegar and water in a spray bottle, add a few drops of your favourite essential oil if you prefer a scent.

Clean and sanitise wood or plastic cutting boards with a lemon! Cut it in half, run it over the surfaces, let sit for ten minutes, and then rinse away.

Dishwasher Soap: 1 cup of liquid castile soap and 1 cup of water (2 teaspoons of lemon juice optional) store in a glass jar and add as required.

Dishwasher Rinse Aid/Glass Cleaner: White vinegar

CHANGE YOUR SUGAR FIX

The history of the discovery of the cigarette – lung cancer link by Dr. Robert.N.Proctor, Stanford University: tobaccocontrol.bmj.com/content/21/2/87

Dietary Fats, Carbohydrates and Artherosclerotic Vascular Disease by McGandy RB, Heysted DM, Stare FJ, *New England Journal of Medicine*, August 1967:
https://nature.berkeley.edu/garbelottoat/wp-content/uploads/Mcgandy-1967-part-2-1.pdf

Discredited by JAMA in 2010:
http://jamanetwork.com/journals/jamainternalmedicine/article-abstract/2548251

Coca-Cola Funds Scientists Who Shift Blame for Obesity Away From Bad Diets by Anahad O'Connor, August 2015:
https://well.blogs.nytimes.com/2015/08/09/coca-cola-funds-scientists-who-shift-blame-for-obesity-away-from-bad-diets/

'Coke tries to sugarcoat the truth on calories', *New York Times*, August 2015:
https://www.nytimes.com/2015/08/14/opinion/coke-tries-to-sugarcoat-the-truth-on-calories.html

ACKNOWLEDGMENTS

I have many people to thank for helping me turn my thoughts, feelings and processes into *Mind Body Miracle*.

Firstly my book coach Wendy Yorke who has mentored me during this cathartic writing process and helped me turn a contents list into a fully-fledged book. Thank you, Wendy, for keeping me accountable and ensuring that my book journey didn't have too many pit stops.

To all the many others who have helped bring this book to fruition. Suzanne Chumbley for photography, Andy King at Glossed and all at Rethink Press. Thank you for your expertise and patience.

To my sister Joanna, who is the only other person in the world who felt the same pain as me at the same time. I know that it has been tough for you to revisit the memories, but that didn't stop you proof reading this book and providing feedback that no-one else could have done. I'm so glad you were brave enough, and delighted it has helped you on your own journey. You are my favourite success story.

To my Soul Garden angels: Katie Brewis, Sarah Wakeling and Joanne Bale. You have no idea how special you make me feel. My heart-centred hippies who dare to dream. You weirdos are my tribe and I love you wildly.

To my countless clients who have brought me many a challenge, you have been my greatest teachers. I thank you for trusting me with your wellbeing and I am so grateful to have been part of your journey and transformation.

To fellow awakened practitioners, healers and light workers – stand strong and speak your truth. You are doing great. Keep going.

To my business partner, contributor and husband, James, thank you for your unconditional love. You have put up with me at times when I could hardly put up with myself. You believed in me before I believed in myself, and you loved me before I loved myself. My teacher, my trigger, my twin flame. I love you.

To my beautiful girls Angelica and Honey. You inspire me to be better, to learn more, to teach more and to bring about change in a world where change is much needed. I feel your impressionable eyes watching me, they inspire me to show you that anything is possible. Every single day you make me proud, my heart is full of love and gratitude for you both. Keep shining, my little stars, and have the courage to follow your dreams.

ACKNOWLEDGMENTS

To Mum and Mamdouh. Thank you for the unconditional love, the kindness, the confidence, the courage, the belief, the wisdom, the teachings, the story, the memories. You told me to go make you proud – so I did.

THE AUTHOR

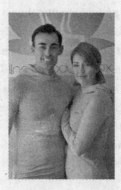

Jaclyn Dunne is a health and nutrition coach as well as a hypnotherapist; she is passionate about holistic healing and the mind-body connection after using the tools laid out in this book to heal her own auto immune condition.

Jaclyn started her working life as an accountant, employed by several big corporations in the City of London across a 17-year period.

She began her journey into health and wellness after a devastating, life-changing experience that made her realise just how short and fragile life can be and served as a stark reminder that she needed to be far more respectful of her own health and life goals.

She has since gained a diploma in hypnotherapy and is a member of the National Hypnotherapy Society. She also gained an advanced diploma in nutritional studies and become a member of the International Institute of Complementary Therapists. She is a member of the CHEK institute, Europe after completing holistic lifestyle coach level one (HLC1).

In 2014 Jaclyn founded the Mind and Body Detox programme, which brings about positive lifestyle changes in health, habits, diet, fitness and mind-set using her knowledge of nutrition and hypnotherapy. She has now helped hundreds of people to gain an understanding and self-belief that enable them to live a healthier and happier life.

If you would like more information on the services provided by Jaclyn, please visit:

www.mindandbodydetox.co.uk
Facebook: Mind and Body Detox
Instagram: mindandbody_detox_jaclyn_dunne